CANNABIS DRINKS

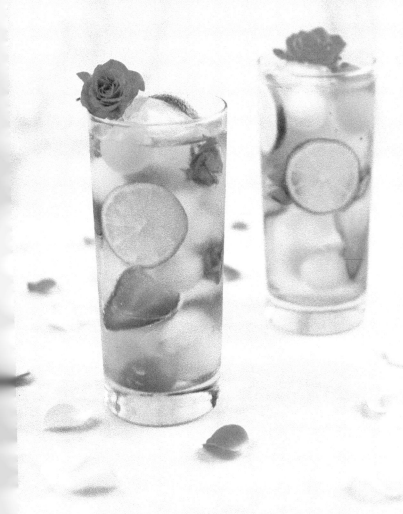

Quarto.com

© 2021 Quarto Publishing Group USA Inc.
Text © 2021 Jamie Evans

Paperback edition published in 2024

First Published in 2021 by Fair Winds Press, an imprint of The Quarto Group,
100 Cummings Center, Suite 265-D, Beverly, MA 01915, USA.
T (978) 282-9590 F (978) 283-2742

Fair Winds Press titles are also available at discount for retail, wholesale, promotional, and bulk purchase. For details, contact the Special Sales Manager by email at specialsales@quarto.com or by mail at The Quarto Group, Attn: Special Sales Manager, 100 Cummings Center, Suite 265-D, Beverly, MA 01915, USA.

ISBN: 978-0-7603-9263-8

Digital edition published in 2021
eISBN: 978-1-63159-918-7

Originally found under the following
Cataloging-in-Publication Data

Evans, Jamie (Founder of The Herb Somm), author.
Cannabis drinks : secrets to crafting CBD and THC beverages at home / Jamie Evans.
ISBN 9781592339747 (hardcover) | ISBN 9781631599187 (ebook)
1. Cannabis drinks. 2. Cookbooks.
LCC TX817.C36 E93 2021 (print) | LCC TX817.C36 (ebook) | DDC 641.337/9--dc23

LCCN 2020038710 (print) | LCCN 2020038711 (ebook)

Design and Page Layout: Laura Klynstra
Photography by Colleen Eversman of 2nd Truth Photography, except pages 52 by Jack Alger; 153 by Boris Bezman; 5, 37, 43, 58, 84, 88, 111, 140 by Jamie Evans; 6, 173 by Chris Greenwell; 71 by Daniel Lee; 157 by Roberto Loppi; 113 by Salina MacKay; 24 by Max Montrose; 18 by Traci Seville; 55 via Shutterstock; 44 by Star Strul; 76 by Vertosa Inc.
Illustrations on pages 29 and 30 by Gilda Harger (except those for humulene, ocimene, terpinolene, via Shutterstock)

To my husband, Stratos.
Thank you for encouraging me to
follow my dreams. I love you.

CANNABIS DRINKS

Secrets to Crafting CBD and THC Beverages at Home

JAMIE EVANS

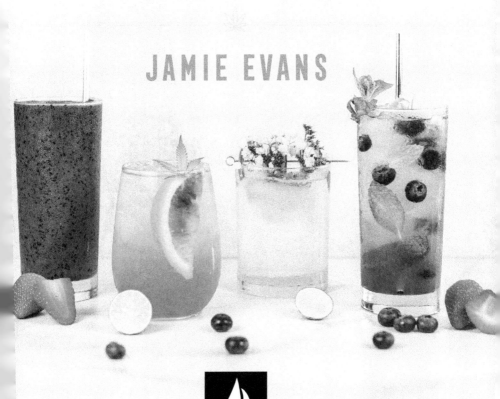

FAIR WINDS

CONTENTS

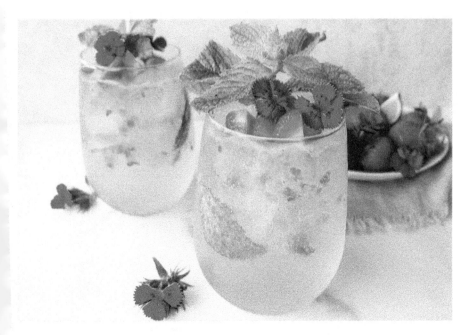

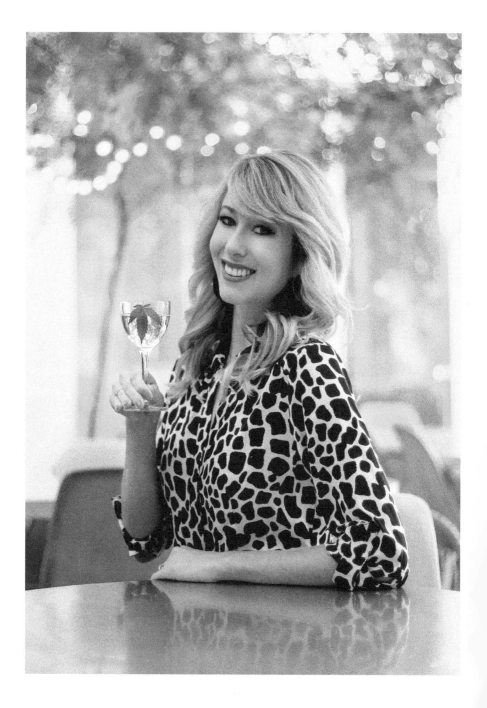

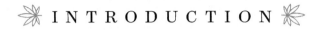 INTRODUCTION

Welcome to the future of beverages.

Infused drinks are one of the fastest growing cannabis categories, quickly becoming the new star of cannabis legalization. From CBD lattes to THC sparkling tonics, consumers can't get enough. There are a number of professionally made products available to experiment with, but crafting cannabis drinks at home has never been easier.

As a Certified Specialist of Wine and a cannabis drink expert, crafting well-made beverages has always been a passion of mine. I fell in love with the gourmet world early on, including all the fanciful drinks that have made their way onto our favorite menus. With my growing interest in food, beverages, flavors, and aromas, it was a natural fit to pursue a career in the wine industry, which I called home for over a decade. Eventually, my love for wine and beverages carried over to cannabis, largely driven by the many similarities between the two. This rings true especially when it comes to infused drinks.

There's something satisfying about creating the perfect melody of aromas and flavors to entice the nose and palate. With the addition of cannabis, we can experience our favorite beverages in an entirely new way. Infused beverages taste great and, by integrating CBD, THC, and an array of other important compounds produced by the cannabis plant, they can also offer many therapeutic benefits.

CBD 101

If you're just beginning your cannabis journey, it's important to familiarize yourself with some basics. Before diving into CBD, let's begin with something called hemp. To clarify, cannabis and hemp are the same plant. When you hear the term "hemp," it's used to classify varieties of cannabis that contain no more than 0.3 percent THC by dry weight, delivering no intoxicating effects when consumed.

However, not all hemp plants are grown the same way. There are different levels of quality within the category. To receive the most therapeutic value from hemp, choose full-spectrum items that are sourced from hemp farms using regenerative farming practices, not big industrial hemp farms. Most often industrial hemp is grown for hemp seed oil or for fiber, not for phytocannabinoid and terpene production, which are the critical components that contribute to the plant's special healing benefits, including CBD.

So, what is CBD, anyway? As one of the most popular phytocannabinoids—meaning a cannabinoid that is derived from a plant—CBD is a nonintoxicating and nonaddicting organic compound that's created by the cannabis plant. Produced in trichomes (the special glands that create the wonderful components that make cannabis unique), CBD works with hundreds of other important compounds to deliver beneficial effects.

While research on CBD and its healing benefits are still in the early stages, there are a few things we do have a reasonable understanding of. For example, while CBD does not deliver the same "high" effects as THC, it can help relieve anxiety and stress by interacting with serotonin receptors found in the brain. CBD is also a powerful anti-inflammatory, inhibiting the release of signaling molecules that come from immune cells that promote inflammation in the body. This is one reason cannabidiol is popular among athletes!

Unlike THC, CBD will not make you feel "stoned." In fact, you might not perceive any noticeable effects at first because CBD is very subtle. As you will learn throughout this book, to achieve the best results with CBD, you must stick with a daily regimen based on your particular needs. Cannabidiol is a personalized medicine that is most impactful when taken consistently over time.

It's also important to remember that CBD is not a cure-all. Don't let marketing schemes fool you! While CBD can be a beneficial phytocannabinoid and is showing potential to help aid several ailments, CBD will not fix everything and it's not for everyone. If you're someone with a serious health condition such as cancer, I highly recommend speaking to a health care professional before using CBD. CBD is a potent inhibitor of two types of P450 liver enzymes that break down more than a third of prescription drugs. If you're using CBD with a drug that is metabolized by these enzymes, the drug could stay in your system longer, which might be dangerous for your health (especially if consumed at higher doses).

Another common misconception is that CBD is "nonpsychoactive." Due to how CBD interacts with different receptors, such as serotonin 5-HT1A, CBD does affect your brain in some capacity. Instead of using "nonpsychoactive," a better term to use would be "nonintoxicating" as it will not cause a "high" like THC.

WHAT ABOUT THC?

Now that you know more about CBD, let's talk about THC. THC (aka delta-9-tetrahydrocannabinol in its active form) is the primary phytocannabinoid that's created when THCA, THC's nonintoxicating acidic precursor found in raw cannabis, is exposed to heat. Found in several variations, THC delivers the "high" or euphoric effects associated with cannabis, but it can also provide a wealth of therapeutic benefits. Having a strong affinity to binding to CB1 and CB2 receptors found throughout the body in our "endocannabinoid system" (ECS), THC has been known to help aid a broad range of ailments.

Recreationally, THC is enjoyable when consumed properly, but similar to CBD, it's not for everyone: Always take precautions before using products that contain THC. Don't mix with other medications. If you have a serious health condition, be sure to speak with your health care provider before using it.

Start low, go slow.

As you work your way through this book, you'll notice that all of the recipes contain a ratio of CBD *and* THC. There's an important reason for this. Research indicates that due to how CBD works with our ECS it is more effective when combined with even a small amount THC and the other beneficial phytocannabinoids to create a phenomenon known as the "entourage effect."

Introduced in 1998 by Professor Shimon Ben-Shabat and Professor Raphael Mechoulam, the entourage effect has become a pillar in cannabis research. It was discovered that phytocannabinoids such as CBD and THC, when combined with organic compounds known as terpenoids (aka terpenes) and flavonoids, work "in concert" or work as an "entourage" in a beneficial way, interacting with receptors found in the body. It's as if this plant was made for us to consume, which is exemplified by the nature of the ECS.

All humans and mammals have an ECS that helps maintain homeostasis. This biological system is composed of different endocannabinoids (cannabinoids naturally produced by the body), cannabinoid receptors, and enzymes that are expressed throughout the body. With the discovery of the ECS, researchers realized phytocannabinoids, such as CBD and THC, can stimulate these same receptor sites, keeping our systems in check by regulating appetite, mood, memory, inflammation, and more.

Researchers also discovered that our bodies can experience endocannabinoid deficiencies, which can greatly affect our health. To restore homeostasis, cannabis can be used as a supplement to rebalance the ECS. By consuming *both* CBD and THC, this power team delivers the most impactful results. You shouldn't feel like you have to choose one or the other. You can actually embrace both, but with a ratio that works best for you and your individual needs.

BRINGING IT TOGETHER IN THE GLASS

Now for the fun part: cannabis drinks! As the ultimate resource for those who are interested in incorporating phytocannabinoids into a variety of recipes, this guidebook features the most essential how-tos and mixology tips for the canna-curious. Whether you're a beginner or an expert, you'll find a range of options for enhancing your drinks—from simply adding commercially made CBD or THC tinctures to crafting low-dose DIY infusions, such as infused simple syrups, shrubs, and bitters.

For beginners who are sensitive to THC, or are nervous about trying it, I encourage you to start with a commercially made, unflavored cannabis-derived CBD tincture found at licensed dispensaries that contains a 20:1 (pronounced twenty to one) or 18:1 ratio of CBD to THC, which will have minimal intoxicating effects. But because cannabis-derived products are not available everywhere quite yet, using your favorite unflavored hemp-derived full-spectrum tincture will also work.

For those of you who'd rather create your own DIY infusions at home, there are many options to explore to create the most flavorful and well-crafted drinks possible. This is my preferred method for infusing drinks and what's recommended throughout the book.

Offering a deep dive into terpenes, this book also covers my signature techniques for evaluating cannabis aroma and flavor profiles to create perfect flavor pairings. Using sensory evaluation techniques, you'll be able to fine-tune your senses to craft infused beverages at home.

Are you ready to get started? I hope you enjoy this exciting exploration of cannabis drinks!

Cheers,

JAMIE EVANS, *The Herb Somm*

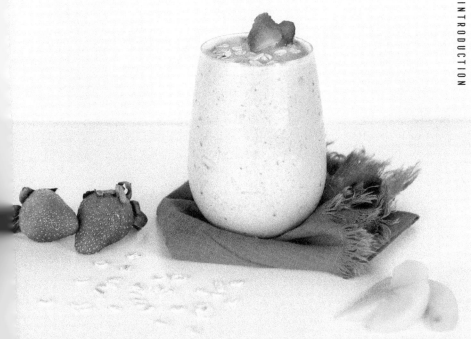

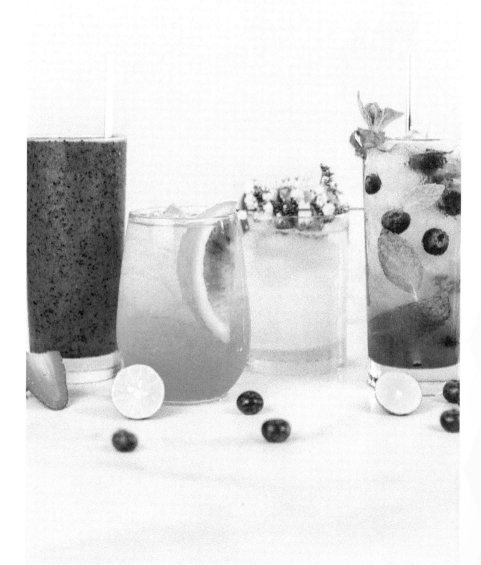

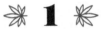

INFUSED BEVERAGE BASICS

There's an art to crafting a delicious drink. When it comes to making cannabis-infused beverages, mixologists and enthusiasts alike are tasked with the heightened challenge of inviting an ensemble of phytocannabinoids and terpenes to enhance a drink's profile. While working with these new, exciting ingredients might seem intimidating at first, once you learn the secrets to crafting infused beverages, you can easily master mixing up cannabis-infused drinks at home.

Let's begin by exploring the basics. These pages highlight the essentials you should know when creating cannabis beverages, including an inside look at how infused drinks interact with your body, an in-depth look into interpreting cannabis aromas and flavors, a guide to dosing, and an overview of how to serve infused drinks properly. Whether you're a fan of nonintoxicating CBD or euphoric THC, understanding these initial concepts will set you up for success as you work your way through this book. Let's dig in!

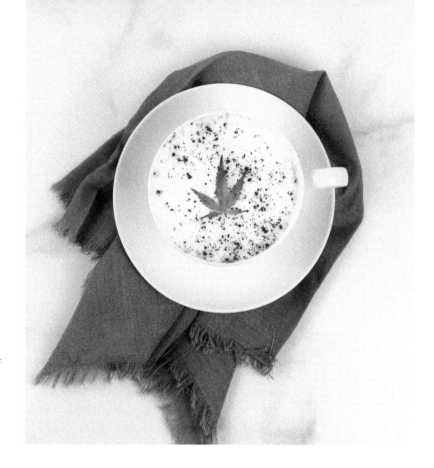

CANNABIS DRINKS 101

By now, you might have noticed that a vast selection of commercially made cannabis-infused drinks have entered the market. If you're new to this category, cannabis-infused beverages can be classified as drinks that've been infused with phytocannabinoids such as CBD or THC. Now available in low-dose options, cannabis-infused drinks are becoming more accessible for casual enjoyment. However, as with all ingestible cannabis items, moderation is key.

NOTE: *You will usually not find alcohol mixed with prepackaged drinkables, even though there's a growing trend of crafting cannabis cocktails at home.*

WORKING WITH CBD AND THC

CBD is a great place to start if you're brand new to cannabis beverages, especially if you're crafting your own drinks and intend to serve them to others. Because CBD is a nonintoxicating phytocannabinoid, you don't have to worry about getting "high" if you accidentally dose the drink inaccurately. When consumed, CBD presents very mild side effects, delivering subtle notes of relaxation. You will not feel a head change or high after consuming CBD, so for some it can be useful during the daytime to help restore balance. However, others may find that CBD can make them feel tired or drowsy.

How cannabidiol impacts you depends on your endocannabinoid system. Before making your first CBD-infused drink, I recommend experimenting with different types of CBD products to gauge how it will make you feel. Once you know how your body handles cannabidiol, you can then make your own CBD beverages and determine what time of day is best for you to consume them.

Personally, I treat CBD like a vitamin and enjoy taking it during the daytime. My CBD routine begins in the morning by adding a teaspoon of CBD honey to my tea or smoothie, or a ¼ cup (60 ml) of CBD-infused milk to my coffee. As the day progresses, I supplement with a CBD tincture or sip on a CBD latte to help me feel balanced throughout the afternoon.

If you're looking to add THC, it's best to first familiarize yourself with the nuances between these two phytocannabinoids. THC is an intoxicating phytocanna-binoid that will make you high. Delivering euphoric side effects, products that contain THC are more noticeable when consumed as compared to CBD. THC presents stronger side effects due to its ability to bind directly to our CB1 and CB2 receptors found throughout the body. While some people feel calm and centered using THC, others might feel waves of paranoia and anxiety if too much is consumed.

When adding THC in any form to beverages, always remember: start low and go slow. Take precautions when working with this powerful phytocannabinoid, but don't be afraid to experiment if you do so wisely.

For me, THC works best at night when I am looking to relax, unwind, and check out from the stressors that may have come up throughout the day. During the work week, I enjoy making low-dose THC (spirit-free) mixed drinks to enjoy before dinner in place of an alcoholic drink. Many have found it can be a great substitute, especially if you're looking to avoid a hangover.

While CBD and THC have their individual characteristics, you shouldn't feel like you have to pick one or the other. The truth is the best drinkable products contain a blend of different phytocannabinoids that enhance each other. Remember the entourage effect (page 10) means a combination of CBD and THC can work together to deliver enhanced therapeutic effects.

I recommend using cannabis flower containing both CBD and THC to craft infusions that will be mixed into a variety of drink recipes. You can also simply use CBD-rich hemp flower or an unflavored full-spectrum CBD or THC tincture to enhance the drinks. If you're looking to avoid THC altogether, you can use broad spectrum hemp-derived CBD to infuse the recipes as well, where THC has been removed from the product completely. Depending on your needs, you can determine what method works best.

UNDERSTANDING BIOAVAILABILITY RATES

Bioavailability refers to the degree and the rate at which a substance is absorbed into the bloodstream. If you're new to the cannabis world, it's important to understand the concept of bioavailability rates, particularly with CBD, to help you determine how much you need to consume, and in what form, to ensure an ideal dose ends up in your system.

When ingested, only a fraction of the CBD you consume will actually affect your body due to a phenomenon known as the *first pass effect*. The first pass effect occurs when a medication, in this case CBD, is greatly reduced in concentration after being metabolized, decreasing its effectiveness after it passes through the gut and liver before reaching the bloodstream. Knowing this, CBD products that are ingested orally and metabolized (i.e., edibles and capsules) tend to have lower bioavailability rates, ranging between 6 and 20 percent, as compared to products that are not ingested (i.e., smokables, transdermal patches, and suppositories) that fall between 30 and 80 percent bioavailable.

While cannabis-infused drinks are indeed ingested and metabolized, they tend to have higher bioavailability rates than other types of products that fall into the oral consumption category. Phytocannabinoids can be absorbed into the bloodstream through the sublingual gland and oral mucosa if the liquid is in contact with these areas for at least 30 to 60 seconds. However, as nanoemulsion technology (page 19) continues to develop, bioavailability rates and onset times for infused drinks are improving due to the nanoscopic size of the phytocannabinoid particles that can be more readily absorbed by the body. It's important to understand these concepts, especially as you begin to experiment with infused drinks.

While the effects of CBD can be greatly reduced by the liver and gut wall, THC is processed differently. Even though bioavailability rates for THC are affected by the liver, as THC passes through, delta-9-THC is converted to 11-hydroxy-THC, a metabolic derivative of THC and an entirely different compound that's formed by the human body rather than the plant itself. When 11-hydroxy-THC is formed after drinking an infused beverage or eating an edible, *you might feel stronger and more longer-lasting effects* when compared to smoking or vaporizing THC products. If you're not used to consuming edibles and drinkables, this can be overwhelming at first. Be especially careful if you're still learning your optimal dosage. For best results, remember the golden rule: start low and go slow.

UNDERSTANDING ONSET TIMES

If you've ever consumed a cannabis-infused beverage, you might have noticed that effects don't set in right away. This is due to the time it takes for phytocannabinoids to be metabolized and absorbed into the bloodstream. Onset times vary from person to person and are often influenced by metabolism, body weight, and diet. While some people feel effects within 20 minutes after drinking an infused beverage, others might not feel anything for more than an hour. As a rule of thumb, you might start noticing effects between 20 and 45 minutes. While CBD is subtle, THC can be intense. Knowing this, it's very important to be patient when consuming THC. Just because you don't feel the effects right away, do not consume more too soon. If you double down and drink another drink too early, the effects may be twice as strong, easily leading to an uncomfortable experience. Remember to be patient!

CRAFTING CANNABIS-INFUSED, ZERO-PROOF WINE

featuring Cynthia Salarizadeh & Tracey Mason,
co-founders of House of Saka

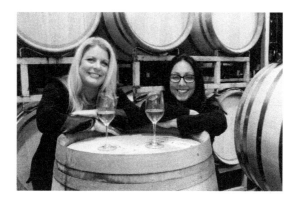

Founded in 2018, Cynthia Salarizadeh and wine industry veteran, Tracey Mason, came together with a mission to create the world's first line of luxury, cannabis-infused products made by and for women. Discovering a shared passion for wine, beauty products, and the boundless properties of the sacred cannabis plant, the pair assembled an unparalleled group of powerful females from both the cannabis and wine industries to help bring their mission to life, creating House of Saka. Look for House of Saka's PINK and WHITE cannabis-infused zero-proof wine and follow their adventures on Instagram @infusedsaka.

CYNTHIA SALARIZADEH & TRACEY MASON: "Making cannabis-infused, nonalcoholic wine that tastes good is no easy feat, but just as with any wine, it all begins with the appellation and the vineyard.

House of Saka wines are made from grapes picked at the peak of ripeness from select vineyards within California's renowned Napa Valley. The grapes are pressed, traditionally fermented, and aged in stainless steel and oak barrels for optimum flavor and aroma development. Once the wine is ready to be bottled, we use a combination of vacuum distillation and reverse osmosis to gently remove the alcohol and replace it with a proprietary, water-soluble THC:CBD formulation.

Natural grape compounds and extracts are used to build back the flavors and textures that are lost when the alcohol is removed. In doing so, makers of cannabis-infused wine seek to create a perfect balance of fruit, acid, and tannins that offer the consumers an authentic wine experience at a fraction of the calories and without the negative effects of alcohol.

Our THC:CBD formulation is created using state-of-the-art nanoemulsion technology that breaks highly refined cannabis oil into nanoscopic particles that are self-homogenizing and highly bioavailable. Because the formulation is immediately absorbed through the mouth and stomach lining rather than through the liver like traditional edibles, the onset effects come on quickly—usually within 5 to 15 minutes— giving the user immediate biofeedback as to how many milligrams is the right dose for them.

A standard 5-ounce (150-ml) glass of Saka PINK or WHITE contains 5 milligrams of THC and 1 milligram of CBD, which we consider a good place to start if you're brand new to cannabis drinks. Considered a low-dose within the cannabis world, this THC to CBD ratio is sensual and relaxing, predictable and consistent. Nanoemulsion technology also supports a rapid dissipation rate, allowing for a highly sessionable, controlled, and truly elevated cannabis experience. Cheers!"

ESSENTIALS FOR ASSEMBLING YOUR OWN CANNABIS DRINKS

Before mastering the art of making infused beverages, you must learn how to work with the cannabis plant itself and evaluate its natural flavors. By understanding the plant's unique characteristics, you can combine CBD or THC infusions with other ingredients to create the perfect exotic elixirs. Once you are comfortable with analyzing terpenes and thoroughly understand the concept of pairing cannabis with ingredients, you can then think about how you'll properly dose your drinks. In this section, you'll learn these principles and more. Let's begin with an exploration of cannabis flower.

CANNABIS FLOWER

The majority of the infusion recipes in chapter 3 call for your choice of decarboxylated cannabis or hemp flower. By selecting a strain that's right for you, you can easily craft cannabis drinks at home.

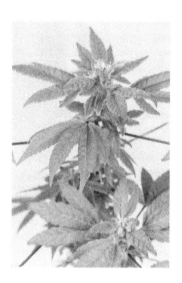

NOTE: *The most effective products are whole-plant derived items that contain a "full spectrum" of CBD, THC, plus other phytocannabinoids, terpenes, flavonoids, and fatty acids. Crafting infusions using flower will ensure that you receive the combined benefits from each unique property.*

When making infused products at home, choose a strain that best suits your needs. Be sure that the flower is clean and pesticide-free. To ensure quality, only source items from a licensed dispensary or a trustworthy resource that can provide you with lab results or a Certificate of Analysis (COA).

If you're looking to create CBD-rich infusions, some CBD to THC ratios to look for include 20:1 (commonly called "twenty to one" though it can also be described as 20% CBD to 1% THC), 18:1, 8:1, 4:1, 3:1 or even 1:1 if you're looking for a more balanced experience.

CBD-Rich Flower Strains

CBD-rich strains can either be classifed as a cannabis (i.e., marijuana) or hemp variety depending on how much THC is in the strain. Some of the most common strains include ACDC, Cannatonic, Charlotte's Web, Harlequin, Harle-Tsu, Sour Tsunami, Haleigh's Hope, Ringo's Gift, Dancehall, Suzy Q, Omrita Rx, Valentine X, Critical Mass, Abacus, Canna-Tsu, and Sour Space Candy. For the recipes in this book, I used Cannatonic for the drink infusions that measured at 12% CBD and 3% THC before decarboxylation.

THC-Rich Flower Strains

If you're a fan of THC, some of the most common cannabis strains that you might come across in a licensed dispensary include OG Kush, Jack Herer, Lemon Haze, Tangie, Blue Dream, Gelato, Sour Diesel, Purple Punch, Kosher Kush, Golden Lemons, and Forbidden Fruit. If you prefer a stronger dose of THC, you can certainly use one of these strains to craft the infusions found in this book. Just be sure to calculate the estimated dosage before consuming or serving to others (see more on page 31).

Balanced Flower Strains

When purchasing cannabis flower, you might also come across cannabis strains that fall somewhere between CBD-rich and THC-rich. These strains contain both CBD and THC, but in a more balanced ratio compared to the other two categories. For example, these strains might present a 1:1 CBD to THC ratio and can include Harmony Rose, Sweet and Sour Widow, and sometimes Cannatonic.

NOTE: *When purchasing cannabis, you might come across items classified as "indica" or "sativa" based on the product's predicted effects. To set the record straight, this is not the most accurate way to determine how cannabis strains will make you feel. When it comes to the classification of indica versus sativa, the distinction between the two is much more relevant to cultivators and plant breeders than to consumers. In fact, the cannabis industry is slowly trying to move away from labeling cannabis products into these two categories because most of what's on the market today is actually a hybrid of the two. What you really need to focus on are phytocannabinoids, and most importantly, terpenes, in order to truly understand how cannabis products will make you feel.*

Evaluating Cannabis: Discovering Terpenes

Much like wine, cannabis is packed with aromas, flavors, and different properties. Each strain has characteristics based on the farming practices and the terroir in which the plant was grown, creating distinctive terpene profiles. Terpenes are the organic compounds that give plants, herbs, flowers, and spices varying aromas, flavors, and therapeutic properties. In cannabis, they are produced in trichomes, the special glands that create phytocannabinoids and all of the other special compounds that make cannabis unique.

Terpenes offer many benefits and can help differentiate strains due to their expressive smells and tastes. Because terpenes interact synergistically with phytocannabinoids to create what researchers call the entourage effect, certain strains make you feel uplifted and energized while others make you feel sleepy and relaxed.

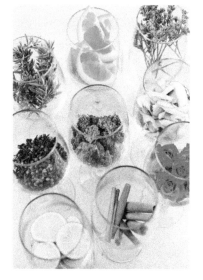

More than 200 terpenes have been identified in cannabis so far, each with its unique aroma and flavor profile. By tapping into your senses, you can recognize the differences between terpenes and apply this knowledge to craft cannabis drinks.

To help identify specific terpenes, here's a look at nine of the most common terpenes along with their aroma and flavor profiles, benefits, and effects. For a listing of my recommended terpene and beverage pairings, flip to page 29.

BETA-CARYOPHYLLENE
Aromas & Flavors: cloves, black pepper, cinnamon, copaiba
Benefits: anti-anxiety, anti-inflammatory, antioxidant, pain reliever
Effects: analgesic, calm, stress free

HUMULENE
Aromas & Flavors: hops, earthy, fresh-cut wood, coriander, cloves
Benefits: anti-inflammatory, antibacterial, appetite suppressant, pain reliever
Effects: euphoric, relaxed, sedated

LIMONENE
Aromas & Flavors: lemon, lime, grapefruit, blood orange, tangerine
Benefits: stress reliever, weight loss aid, mood enhancer
Effects: uplifted, energized

LINALOOL
Aromas & Flavors: lavender, citrus blossoms, violets, roses, lilies
Benefits: anti-anxiety, sleep aid, muscle relaxant, antidepressant, anti-acne
Effects: relaxed, blissful, rejuvenated

MYRCENE
Aromas & Flavors: earthy, mixed herbs, mushrooms, skunk, tropical fruits, mango
Benefits: sleep aid, muscle relaxant, antidepressant
Effects: sleepy, sedated

NEROLIDOL
Aromas & Flavors: jasmine, perfume, ginger flower, tea tree
Benefits: antifungal, antidepressant, sleep aid
Effects: tranquil, peaceful

OCIMENE
Aromas & Flavors: parsley, basil, mint, oregano, tarragon, bergamot, kumquat
Benefits: antioxidant, decongestant, anti-inflammatory
Effects: uplifted, energized

PINENE
Aromas & Flavors: pine trees, pine needles, wet wood, pine nuts, dill, rosemary
Benefits: asthma reliever, provides energy, anti-inflammatory
Effects: alert, focused

TERPINOLENE
Aromas & Flavors: lilac, pine tree, citrus, nutmeg, cumin, allspice, perfume
Benefits: antibacterial, antifungal, antioxidant
Effects: relaxed, sedated

Now that you know some of the most common terpene profiles, let's explore a few sensory evaluation techniques that will help you craft world-class cannabis drinks.

THE ART OF INTERPENING

featuring Max Montrose, founder of the Trichome Institute
& professional cannabis sommelier

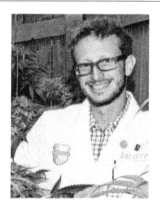

Max Montrose is the founder of the Trichome Institute, the nation's leading educational program that specializes in providing a certifiable cannabis curriculum for professionals and recreational users. As the creator of "interpening" and author of Interpening, Max is known as one of the world's top cannabis sommeliers and continuously researches cannabis to provide the world with proper education about this amazingly complex and beautiful plant. Follow Max @max.montrose and the Trichome Institute @trichome.institute or visit www.TrichomeInstitute.com.

MAX MONTROSE: "If you're looking to take your cannabis education to the next level, interpening is an immersive cannabis sommelier program that dives deep into the science of evaluating cannabis flower to determine quality, variety, type, and psychotropic effects, through physical and aromatic inspection.

Interpening is based on a combination of science, theory, and art, which requires significant experience to master. This program was inspired by the model of the certified wine sommelier, including education, books, and interactive tools. There are now thousands of "Interpeners" worldwide dedicated to this methodology, which is expanding into cannabis appellations, terroir, grading, and so much more.

Learning how to evaluate cannabis is incredibly important because current testing requirements do not include terpene testing to provide insight into possible psychotropic effects. Strain names, speciation terms, cannabinoid content, and the like will not tell you the quality of cannabis flower or how it will make you feel when you consume it. Luckily, interpening will!

So, how does interpening work? By visually evaluating the physical characteristics of the flower and interpreting the aromatics of the terpenes. It will also enable you to identify potential flaws in your flower such as spider mites, improper flushing, etc.

If you're aspiring to be a cannabis sommelier, interpening will teach you the evolution of global cannabis speciation and what to properly call thousands of cultivars. You'll also learn cannabis history, terminology, botany, and functions of the plant, plus how to identify cannabis quality and accurately predict where the cannabis will land on the stimulant to sedative scale. These are essentials for becoming an expert.

I encourage you to join us at the Trichome Institute if you're seeking a higher level of cannabis education. It is our goal to teach you the latest discoveries in cannabis research, giving you the skills that you need to succeed as a certified Interpener."

EXERCISES TO ENHANCE YOUR SENSE OF SMELL FOR CANNABIS

Now that you know some of the basic principles of interpening (see page 24), here are five exercises I recommend to improve your sense of smell for cannabis.

EXERCISE 1: Aroma is closely linked to your memory. As a first step, try to remember past scents and present smells you encounter throughout the day. Creating this awareness will help you remember aromas and flavors later.

EXERCISE 2: Purchase items commonly mentioned in cannabis descriptions, such as lemons, grapefruits, blueberries, mushrooms, lavender, strawberries, and tropical fruits such as mango. Muddle the items, placing them into small jars or wine glasses, and smell the aromas. Remember, what you are smelling are terpenes! You should also take a bite, as the flavors can enhance and help you remember the aromas.

EXERCISE 3: Explore dried herbs and spices. Gather a selection of spices that represent similar aromas that you'd find in cannabis. I recommend rosemary, thyme, black pepper, dill, basil, cinnamon, and clove. Smell each spice separately. Close your eyes, inhale several times briefly, and note what you are smelling. Next, taste the spice and savor it on your palate.

EXERCISE 4: Apply what you've learned to detect different terpene profiles in cannabis. You'll want to smell several different strains in one session. Keep the cannabis in its jar or, if you're at home, transfer the flower to wine glasses and smell the different strains one by one. Do you recognize any familiar scents? If so, you've successfully used your sense of smell to identify terpenes in your cannabis.

EXERCISE 5: The best way to evaluate the flavor is to use a dry flower vaporizer (see Resources on page 170). Or you can use a joint or preroll and use a technique called the "dry pull," meaning you inhale for flavor without lighting the cannabis to evaluate the terpenes. As you taste the flower, make notes and think about what ingredients would pair well with it.

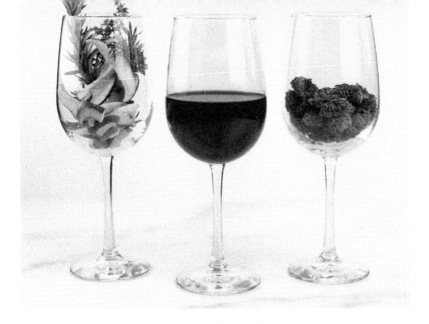

PAIRINGS: THE BITE PHILOSOPHY

As you might have discovered, cannabis products pair exceptionally well with many types of cuisines and beverages. If you're curious to learn how to create the perfect pairings, try following these simple steps, so you can master the art of integrating flavors when mixing up cannabis drinks. I call it the "BITE" philosophy: balance, intention, taste, enjoy.

B: Balance

When pairing cannabis with drinks, the weight of the cannabis strain and the weight of the beverage must be balanced. For cannabis, weight is determined by its effect and potency. For drinks, weight is determined by body and richness. To better understand this concept, think of a bold Cabernet Sauvignon compared to a crisp Sauvignon Blanc. The red wine is more full-bodied and rich on the palate compared to the light-bodied, refreshing white wine. With cannabis, you can use a similar evaluation approach. Heavier, sedating strains that are rich in earthy myrcene, or perhaps spicy beta-caryophyllene, are considered bold and weighty. Lighter, energizing strains with citrusy limonene or minty ocimene are considered light and uplifting. The trick is to keep the cannabis and drink characteristics balanced, so one doesn't overpower the other.

I: Intention

Your intention for the pairing plays a factor in determining the best combinations. How do you want to feel? If you are looking to have a relaxing night at home, a more mellow strain with high levels of myrcene might be the preferred option paired with a glass of Grenache. If you're going out with friends, consider using an energy-boosting strain containing pronounced levels of limonene to feel uplifted and social, perhaps paired with a glass of Champagne. Think about the occasion and your intention to find the perfect match.

T: Taste

The most important factor to consider when pairing is the actual taste of the combination. I recommend getting to know your terpene profiles. You'll also want to learn how to identify aromas and flavors in different drinks and pay close attention to the ingredients you are working with. Think of your cannabis as a sommelier would think about a wine. By comparing or contrasting cannabis terpene aroma and flavor profiles with your favorite drinks or ingredients, you can create the perfect pairings. Remember, the goal when creating a pairing is for the components to enhance each other. You might even be surprised to find that the combination creates an entirely new flavor not yet experienced in the beverage or cannabis alone.

E: Enjoy

The final tip to a successful cannabis pairing is to enjoy it! There are so many incredible pairings out there. The combinations are endless, so find what works best for your personal palate. To help you become a pairing wiz at home, use the Herb Somm pairing guide (opposite) as you explore terpene profiles with a variety of beverage recipes.

	TERPENE AROMAS	CANNABIS STRAINS	BEVERAGE PAIRINGS
Beta-caryophyllene	Cloves, Black Pepper, Cinnamon, Copaiba	Omrita RX, Northern Lights, Dancehall	Spiced Rum, Apple Spice Mule, Pumpkin Spice Canna-Latte, Masala Chai Tea, Zinfandel, Cabernet Sauvignon
Humulene	Hops, Earthy, Fresh-cut Wood, Coriander, Cloves, Cilantro, Cardamom, Sage	Headband, Peppermint Cookies, Gelato, GSC	Beer, Rioja, Cilantro Margarita, Cardamom Apple Shrub Soda, Sage Bee's Knees
Limonene	Lemon, Lime, Grapefruit, Blood Orange, Tangerine	Lemon Haze, OG Kush, Tangie	Limelight, Hot Toddy, Grey-hound, Cranberry Orange Spritz, Margarita, Char-donnay, Albarino, Limoncello
Linalool	Lavender, Citrus Blossoms, Citrus, Violets, Roses, Lilies	Pink Kush, Lavender OG, LA Confidential, Amnesia Haze	Lavender Lemon Collins, Lavender French 75, Rose Cucumber Collins, Spring Queen, Muscat, Riesling, Nebbiolo, Viognier
Myrcene	Earthy, Mixed Herbs, Mushrooms, Forest Floor, Skunk, Tropical Fruits, Mango	Cannatonic, Critical Mass, Harlequin, Harle-Tsu, Pineapple Express	Pinot Noir, Syrah, Grenache, Mango Mule, Pineapple Rum Punch

(continued)

	TERPENE AROMAS	CANNABIS STRAINS	BEVERAGE PAIRINGS
Nerolidol	Jasmine, Perfume, Ginger Flower, Tea Tree, Lemongrass, Floral, Woody	Island Sweet Skunk, Banana Kush, Blue Dream, Royal Cookies	Moscow Mule, Ginger Kombucha, Fuzzy Ginger Fizz, Torrontés, Gewürztraminer
Ocimene	Parsley, Basil, Mint, Oregano, Tarragon, Bergamot, Kumquat	Clementine, Dream Queen, Dutch Treat, Golden Pineapple	Cucumber Tarragon Cooler, Blue Dream Berry Mint Mojito, Sangiovese, Merlot, Pinot Grigio, Kumquat Caipirinha
Pinene	Pine Trees, Pine Needles, Wet Wood, Rosemary, Dill, Parsley, Juniper Berries	ACDC, Jack Herer, Trainwreck, Valentine X	Gin, Bloody Mary, Grapefruit Rosemary Shrub, New Zealand Sauvignon Blanc, Rioja, Rosemary Gimlet
Terpinolene	Lilac, Citrus, Nutmeg, Cumin, Allspice, Perfume, Pine Tree, Sage	Ghost Train Haze, Golden Goat, XJ-13, Orange Cookies	Spiced Sangria, Muscat, Viognier, Pinot Blanc, Allspice Dram, Negroni

HOW TO DOSE INFUSED DRINKS

Now that you've mastered sensory evaluation, it's time to talk about dosing. When crafting cannabis drinks at home, pay close attention to the potency of the product that you're working with. This is crucial, especially if you're working with items or ingredients that contain THC. Consuming CBD alone in an infused beverage will not make you feel "high," but there are still important considerations to remember when crafting infused drinks. Here are my answers to some of the most common questions asked when it comes to dosing beverages.

How Much CBD or THC Is the Goal for a Standard Drink?

If you're planning to infuse drinks solely with CBD, there is no standard for dosing since CBD affects everyone differently. When crafting CBD drinks at home, I recommend starting on the lower side of the dosage range (between 3 to 25 milligrams of CBD). If you're using a commercially made CBD product (i.e., a CBD tincture) to infuse your beverage recipes, most people begin with between 10 to 15 milligrams of CBD per drink. You could also start with the brand's recommended dose per serving and adjust up or down based on your personal preference.

If you're serving others, always stick with a low dose and check in with your guests on what their dosage preferences are. Remember, CBD by itself does not present any intoxicating side effects, so you or your guests will not get high after consuming it in a beverage. Finally, always consult with a health care provider before mixing CBD with other medications, which is typically not recommended.

When working with THC, keep in mind that you should start low and go slow. I recommend experimenting with between 1 to 5 milligrams of THC per beverage, which is a safe place to start if you're a beginner. If you're brand new to THC, never drink a second infused beverage just because you don't feel immediate effects. It's better to try changing the dose and re-making the drink on another day than to accidentally overserve yourself or your guests!

For the more experienced cannabis consumer, if you'd like to have a sessionable cannabis drink experience (i.e., drink more than one), it's best to stick to a low dosage so you can have a second or third drink in one sitting and still be comfortable. As you work your way through this book, the recipes demonstrate this low-dose approach.

Important: The cannabis drink DIY infusions in this book have been crafted to accommodate low to medium CBD and THC dosing. If you're someone who requires a high dose, luckily you can easily use a commercially made high-potency tincture to best suit your needs or turn to page 70 to learn how to increase the potency of the DIY infusions featured. Always remember to use precautions when testing new commercially made products as they vary across the board.

Can You Taste CBD or THC When They're Added to Drinks?

The "taste" of the CBD or THC depends on how you craft the beverage and what type of products you use to enhance the drink. If you infuse cannabis flower into a mixer such as simple syrup, you might taste some herbaceous notes, but this flavor is often softened by the other ingredients. If you're simply adding commercially made CBD or THC oil drops to the drink, you may taste it as well, but dosing is more accurate because the amount of CBD or THC is listed on the packaging. If you're new to cannabis or infused beverages, the precision of manufactured products can be valuable, especially for those sensitive to THC. To ensure you're using a clean product, look for a Certificate of Analysis (COA) and lab results, especially when it comes to hemp-derived CBD as these items are not thoroughly tested.

While some cannabis mixologists prefer an herbal taste, others try to mask cannabis's flavor. It depends on your palate and taste preferences, but for the purposes of this book, I will teach you how to complement it!

Are There Any Risks When Creating Cannabis Drinks?

If you're taking prescription medication, it is not recommended to mix with CBD or THC. CBD can either enhance or inhibit the way some medications interact with your body. If you're thinking about using cannabis for the first time, it's imperative that you speak with your health care provider to limit the risk of potentially dangerous drug interactions if you're on other medications. If your primary doctor is not familiar with cannabinoid medicine, other resources can guide you including the American Cannabinoid Clinics or a cannabis coach, such as Dr. Michele Ross, who consults international clients who are curious about exploring plant-based medicines.

Until you're familiar with the effects of consuming an infused beverage, limit consumption and experiment cautiously. Always keep track of your milligram intake—especially if you are drinking THC-infused beverages.

HOW TO DOSE CANNABIS DRINKS USING HANDCRAFTED INFUSIONS

Dosing and accurately measuring the potency of an enhanced drink can be tricky when crafting infusions at home, due to the nature of the DIY infusion process. Luckily, you can follow the steps below to estimate the potency of the beverages you'll be creating using handcrafted infusions. For best results, I always recommend carefully evaluating each new infusion for potency before incorporating it into your recipes by sampling ¼ to ½ teaspoon of the infusion first.

The Dosage Calculation

This formula can be used to calculate the final amount of CBD and THC per serving, based on different liquid infusion bases.

STEP 1: Determine how much total CBD or THC is in your dry flower after you purchase it.

To estimate the total amount of CBD and THC that will be in your infusion, combine CBD + CBDA and THC + THCA percentages to determine the potency. This information should be listed on the packaging of the flower when you purchase it. Multiply the CBDA or THCA by a 0.877 conversion rate and add it to your CBD and THC to get your total CBD and total THC. If CBDA and THCA percentages are not listed on the packaging, then this conversion has most likely already been done for you.

Example: For the recipes in this book, I used Cannatonic that measured at 12 percent CBD and 3 percent THC before decarboxylation (CBDA and THCA were already converted over).

STEP 2: Convert CBD and THC percentages to determine milligrams per gram of dry flower (1 gram = 1,000 milligrams).

Example: Based on the starting values in Step 1, 12 percent CBD and 3 percent THC

0.12 x 1,000 mg/g = 120 mg CBD per gram of dry flower
0.03 x 1,000 mg/g = 30 mg THC per gram of dry flower

STEP 3: After you decarboxylate the flower, account for loss during the heating process if you're using an oven (33 percent estimated when using a standard oven to decarb).

Example: Remaining after 33 percent loss

120 mg/g x 0.67 = 80.4 mg/g CBD
30 mg/g x 0.67 = 20.1 mg/g THC

STEP 4: Multiply the remaining CBD and THC from Step 3 by grams of flower called for in your recipe.

Example: For infused milk, the recipe calls for 3.5 grams of cannabis flower

80.4 mg/g x 3.5 grams = 281.40 mg CBD
20.1 mg/g x 3.5 grams = 70.35 mg THC

STEP 5: Convert your primary infusion base (i.e., water, milk, etc.) into grams. To make the conversions easy, here is a quick conversion guide.

Example: 3 cups milk = 765 grams

INGREDIENT	SERVING SIZE	GRAMS
Water	1 cup (8 ounces)	240
Milk	1 cup (8 ounces)	255
Whiskey, Vodka, Rum, Gin	1 cup (8 ounces)	235
Everclear	1 cup (8 ounces)	216

STEP 6: When heating your flower infusions for longer periods of time, you must account for loss due to evaporation. Use the chart following to calculate the remaining volume (or final yield) of your ingredient after loss. If you did not heat the infusion (i.e., when making a heat-free alcohol tincture), skip this step.

Example: After you account for the percentage loss, you have your final yield

765 grams of milk x 0.875 = 669.38 (final yield), assuming 12.5% loss during infusion process

INGREDIENT	% LOSS OF VOLUME DURING INFUSION PROCESS
Milk	12.5% (Heating 1 Hour)
Water (Simple Syrup)	12.5% (Heating 1 Hour)
Alcohol	12.5% - 25% (Heating 1 to 2 hours)

STEP 7: Determine the number of servings remaining in your final yield. Divide your answer from Step 6 by the number of grams per serving, indicated in the chart below.

Example: Based on the final yield from Step 6

669.38 grams / (28 grams of infused milk per ounce) = 23.9 ounces

INGREDIENT	SERVING SIZE	GRAMS
Milk	1 ounce	28
Simple Syrup	1 ounce	28
Alcohol Tinctures	1 milliliter	0.789

STEP 8: Finally, divide your remaining CBD and THC from Step 4 by the number of servings in Step 7. This gives you CBD and THC per serving.

Example: Final calculation for infused milk

281.40 mg / 23.9 ounces = 11.77 or 12 mg CBD per ounce (30 ml) of infused milk
70.35 mg / 23.9 ounces = 2.94 or 3 mg THC per ounce (30 ml) of infused milk

HOW TO SERVE INFUSED DRINKS

Now that you've mastered dosing, the next step to crafting infused drinks is learning how to serve them safely and responsibly. Here is a checklist of some of the essential dos and don'ts.

DO

Dose each drink individually to ensure consistent, safe consumption.

Ensure that your guests are not taking other medications that might be altered by CBD or other phytocannabinoids—communication is key.

Always clearly state how many milligrams of CBD and THC are in each serving/drink.

Label everything, especially your home-crafted infusions and their potency levels.

Be flexible and willing to accommodate dosage preferences when serving others.

Communicate with your guests to remind them that the beverages are infused.

Keep track of the cumulative amount of CBD or THC milligrams served and consumed.

For formal gatherings, tray pass the infused beverages so your serving staff can relay how many milligrams are in each drink.

DON'T

Overserve your guests.
Remember, start low, go slow to avoid uncomfortable situations.

Infuse large batches of drinks, such as punch, with phytocannabinoids, particularly THC.
Dosing large batches is very inaccurate, and things can go wrong very quickly if your guests consume too much THC. For best results, stick to dosing one drink at a time.

Judge others or assume their dosage preferences.
Remember, everyone is different. Be open to accommodating requests.

Forget to label what is what.
Label, label, label! If you don't, you might accidentally serve someone an infused beverage even though they don't want one.

Serve multiple infused drinks in a row to new consumers, especially if you're serving THC drinks.
Moderation is the key to serving cannabis drinks—don't overdo it.

Above all, it's crucial to remind your guests to be patient when consuming infused beverages. If you follow this checklist, you should avoid the pitfalls when serving cannabis drinks. Consume wisely and serve responsibly!

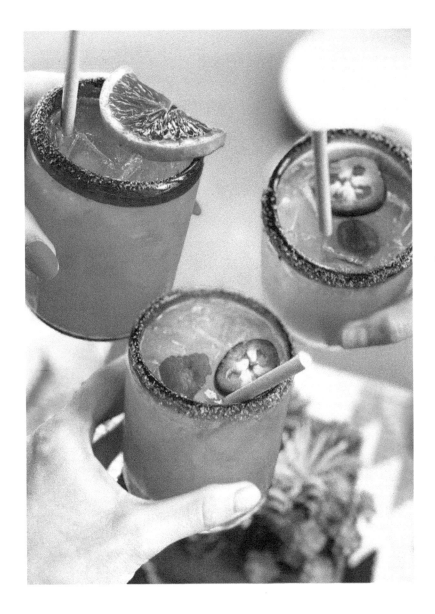

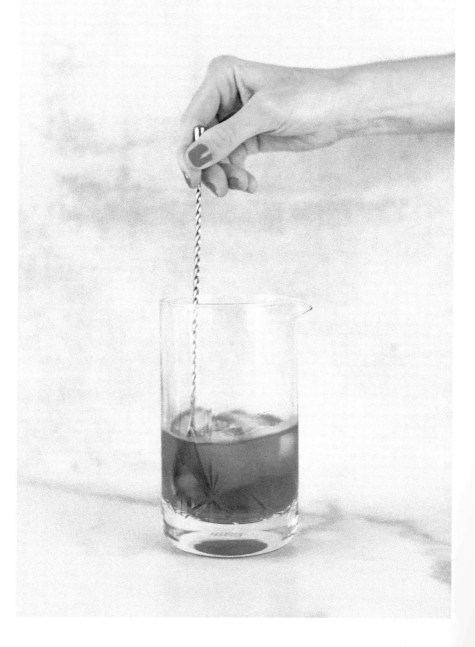

CHAPTER

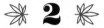

MASTERING MIXOLOGY

If you're new to mixology, consider this chapter your crash course. To create the most delicious cannabis beverages possible, you must master a few important concepts. One of the most important is balance. Is the drink too sweet or too sour? Is it complex or simple? What's the texture like? How can you make this drink more intriguing and palatable?

If these questions are making your head spin, don't worry! With some practice and patience, you'll be able to effortlessly blend ingredients to craft drink recipes that harmonize on your palate. It's just a matter of using the right techniques, sourcing fresh ingredients, and learning to refine the way you taste. Welcome to cannabis mixology 101.

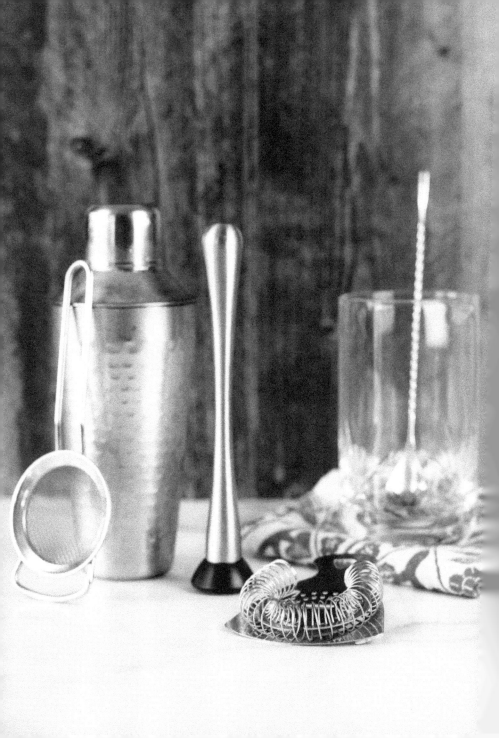

MIXOLOGY TIPS

Mixology is defined as the skill of mixing cocktails and other drinks, but at its core, it's the extensive study of the art and craft of combining flavors. Many of the top mixologists across the country are known for their imaginative and innovative drinks that go far beyond the typical cocktail list. I consider mixologists the alchemists of drinks. Every ingredient that goes into the beverage is meant to enhance the complexity, structure, mouthfeel, and backbone. While it might take years to perfect multidimensional drinks, there's nothing stopping you from putting on your "mixologist hat" and learning how to mix cannabis-infused ingredients into various beverages.

TASTING NOTES ARE KEY

If you've ever been to a wine tasting, you know that an essential step to evaluating a wine is determining its tasting notes. By using sensory evaluation techniques (i.e., using your nose and palate to decipher the characteristics of a wine), you can create tasting notes for any ingredient that you're working with, including cannabis. Before crafting cannabis infusions and drinks, think about your ingredients. Smell and taste each ingredient separately and write down your tasting notes before combining them. What characteristics are you trying to highlight? Focus on this as you build the drink and combine ingredients that accentuate the specific profile that you're aiming for.

CHOOSE QUALITY INGREDIENTS

Similar to cooking, you'll want to choose quality ingredients for your cannabis drinks. If you start with inferior items, such as bruised or old fruit, your drinks will reflect that. For spirit-free mixed drinks and cocktails, choose fresh ingredients over frozen or processed juices if possible. For smoothies, using frozen fruit works best, but be sure the fruit is not packed with added sugar. This thought process can also be applied to the cannabis flower that you'll be using to craft your infusions or the commercially made cannabis oil or tincture that you mix into the drink. Don't use old cannabis or low-quality CBD or THC items that haven't been tested. Be smart and source your products from trustworthy brands and retailers.

DON'T MASK THE FLAVOR OF CANNABIS, COMPLEMENT IT

Many infused oils and tinctures have a pronounced herbaceous taste. Knowing this, I recommend not trying to mask the flavor of cannabis, but complement it instead. One of the best ways to do this is by incorporating terpene-inspired ingredients often found in cannabis's aroma and flavor profiles. Some of the best ingredients include citrus (more on this in a moment!), tropical fruits, mint, lavender, cinnamon, black pepper, mixed herbs, fresh dill, and sometimes ingredients with savory, earthy flavors. Refer to page 29 for a full terpene and aroma guide.

YOU CAN USE EXOTIC INGREDIENTS, BUT NOT TOO MANY

When crafting drinks, particularly cocktails, it might be tempting to add a ton of different liqueurs, shrubs, juices, bitters, and more. While adding exotic ingredients can taste great, more does not mean better. When mixing drinks, remember that your base ingredient should be the star of the show. To add complexity and dimension to your drink, add modifiers (aka fortified wines, liqueurs, shrubs, bitters, and so on), but with moderation. The modifiers should enhance the drink, not overcomplicate it.

CONSIDER COLOR

There's a difference between presenting a cocktail with a bright, beautiful hue and serving up a brown, murky liquid. Regardless if the drink tastes out-of-this-world delicious, if the color is off-putting it will not show well. While it might take some experimentation, combine ingredients that will enhance each color, not take away from it.

TO UP YOUR CANNABIS DRINK GAME, USE FRESH CITRUS

Using fresh citrus in recipes will automatically up your cannabis drinks game. Citrus combines seamlessly with cannabis aromas and flavors, and it can add freshness, tartness, and lively acidity that play well with other ingredients such as sugar and alcohol. When necessary, filter out the pulp using a fine-mesh strainer before mixing with your other ingredients.

SHAKE OR STIR?

Deciding whether to shake or stir is an essential step when considering the drink's mouthfeel. Mouthfeel can be described as the physical sensations in the mouth that are produced by the drink. Is the drink creamy? Silky smooth? Chewy? These are all common descriptors that are used to categorize mouthfeel.

Remember this rule: non-citrus drinks that are primarily made with spirits and liqueurs should be stirred whereas drinks that contain citrus should be shaken. If you're planning to stir, put ice into your mixing glass first, then add the ingredients. Stir the drink in smooth circular motions, keeping your bar spoon even, limiting the oxygen that enters the glass. But if you're making a citrus-forward drink, use a shaker tin to mix the ingredients. The oxygen that's added will liven up your citrus, creating an almost spritzy effect on the palate. Shaking is also great for dairy drinks or recipes that contain egg whites to add a creamy effect.

DON'T FORGET TO GARNISH

Last but not least, don't forget to garnish your drinks! Most times, garnishes will be the first thing your senses encounter when you take the first sip of a beverage, so the aromatics of the garnish are important. Use visually appealing items that complement the rest of the ingredients in the drink and add a pop of color. For bonus points, add something edible, but sometimes a simple wheel of citrus is all you need to top off the perfect cannabis libation. Have fun with it!

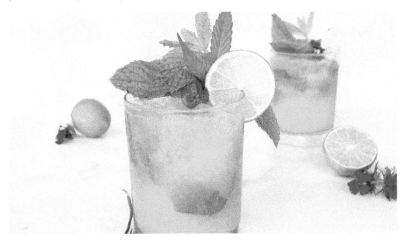

EXOTIC ELIXIRS: EXPLORING CBD AND NOOTROPICS

featuring Maya Elisabeth, owner & founder of Om

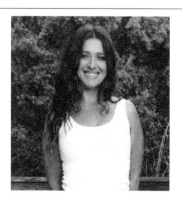

Maya Elisabeth is the owner and founder of Om, a female-operated legacy cannabis company in Berkeley, California. Established in 2008 under the collective model and proposition 215, Om is a "formulation forward" brand, producing thirty different award-winning products including hemp-derived CBD products available worldwide. Maya views cannabis as a superfood, and believes that when cannabis is combined with other superfoods and nutrient-dense ingredients, superior products are made. To learn more, follow Maya and Om at @omedibles or visit www.omedibles.org.

MAYA ELISABETH: "Just like cannabis, nootropics are getting a lot of focus for being cognitive enhancers that support the mind, body, and spirit. Because the government's patent for cannabinoids, CBD in particular, is for antioxidative and neuroprotective properties, combining nootropics and CBD in a drink can provide palpable relaxation and stress relief while enhancing memory and creativity. These powerful allies can take the edge off anxiety, uplift the mood, calm the nerves, decrease inflammation, and taste delicious, all while generating new brain growth and improving memory. Many times these drinks can accomplish the same relieving qualities as alcohol and powerful pharmaceuticals, but instead of having negative side effects, they bring positive health benefits that are non-habit-forming.

Combining both cannabinoids and nootropics, it's my pleasure to present the Psylo-BAE. This drink celebrates our medical plant rights and birthrights to use all plants, especially those that interact with our body's natural receptors. This delicious infused drink is about taking wellness into our own hands and celebrating the many forms of medicine the earth has given us, including mushrooms. Similar to cannabis, mushrooms are incredibly beneficial for our bodies. Enjoy!"

PSYLO-BAE

YIELD: 2 servings

TARGET DOSE: your preferred dose (using Om CBD Elixir or your favorite commercially made CBD or THC tincture)

EQUIPMENT
Shaker tin
Hawthorne strainer

INGREDIENTS
6 ounces (180 ml) pomegranate juice
6 ounces (180 ml) cranberry juice
1 tablespoon (15 ml) aquafaba
1 milliliter Lion's Mane tincture (or your preferred dose)
Om CBD Elixir or your favorite CBD or THC tincture at your preferred dose
Pulverized freeze-dried raspberries, for garnish

Combine all of the ingredients in a shaker tin with ice. Shake vigorously to create as much foam as possible, then strain the liquid into two chilled glasses. Dust the top of each glass with pulverized freeze-dried raspberries to create a toadstool or Amanita muscaria appearance.

BEVERAGE TERMINOLOGY

As you fine-tune your mixology skills, it's important to know the language of making craft drinks.

Alcohol by Volume "ABV": The percentage of alcohol in a bottle of spirits, liquor, wine, or beer.

Aperitif: A drink served before a meal to stimulate the appetite.

Batching: Mixing a large quantity of a drink before serving to a group.

Digestif: A drink served after dinner to help aid digestion.

Dry Shake: Shaking ingredients in a shaker tin without ice.

Fizz: A carbonated beverage that can also contain egg white.

Muddling: A technique used to release oils or juices in a glass by gently pressing ingredients such as mint, limes, or berries with a muddler tool.

On the Rocks: A spirit or mixed drink served in a glass over ice.

Rickey: Typically a gin drink with fresh lime juice, soda water, and sweetener.

Shaking: A technique to chill and mix ingredients, usually in a cocktail shaker tin.

Shrub: Fruit liqueur made with rum or brandy, mixed with sugar and citrus juice or a vinegar-based syrup often mixed with spirits, water, or carbonated water. In this book, you'll create cannabis-infused shrubs with vinegar.

Sour: A drink blend of a base liquor (or a spirit-free cannabis-infused base), lemon/lime juice, and sugar.

Stirring: Using a bar spoon to combine ingredients in a mixing glass filled with ice.

Straight Up: A drink served without ice.

Toddy: A drink typically made of liquor, hot water, sugar, lemon, and spices.

Zero-Proof: A beverage that does not contain alcohol.

MIXING CBD AND THC INTO DRINKS

As you get more comfortable working with infused products and crafting infusions at home, you'll quickly learn there are many ways you can create an infused beverage that go beyond simply adding a commercially made cannabis tincture or CBD oil into your recipe. Using these advanced infusion techniques will help you go the extra mile to craft personalized cannabis-infused drinks. Here are the most common ways to mix CBD and THC into a variety of beverages.

INFUSIONS

One of the best ways to craft cannabis-infused drinks is by creating a selection of infusions that can be easily combined with other beverage ingredients. As important bar pantry items, the infusions featured in this book include honey, simple syrup, shrubs, bitters, and sour mix. If you're new to creating an infusion, it is a process of extracting organic compounds (THC and CBD) from cannabis by using a solvent such as alcohol, oil, butter, or other fat-based liquids. Most professional cannabis mixologists create their own CBD or THC infusions using heating methods such as sous vide, stovetop, slow cooker, or an infusion device. If you're using high-proof alcohol as your solvent (i.e., Everclear), you can also use a non-heating method that combines cannabis flower with alcohol in a Mason jar, then storing the blend in a dark pantry or freezer for a few weeks to create a potent infusion. In the next chapter, you'll use a variety of methods, plus learn how to make delectable infusions that will be used to elevate the drink recipes found in this book.

ALCOHOL OR OIL TINCTURES

One of the easiest ways to add CBD or THC into a drink is using a few drops of a commercially made tincture. One major benefit of this method is precise dosing, compared to using a homemade infusion where you will calculate an estimate of how many milligrams of CBD or THC are in each serving. Remember that alcohol-based tinctures work better than oil-based because they do not separate from liquids. However, some cannabis mixologists prefer using CBD or THC oil for certain drink recipes as it can add a thicker mouthfeel and pleasant complexity (see recipe on page 127) or acts as a decorative garnish. It's up to you to decide what method you'd like to use; however, I recommend alcohol-based tinctures if you're looking to create a drink that integrates well. Turn to page 79 to learn how to make your own tinctures.

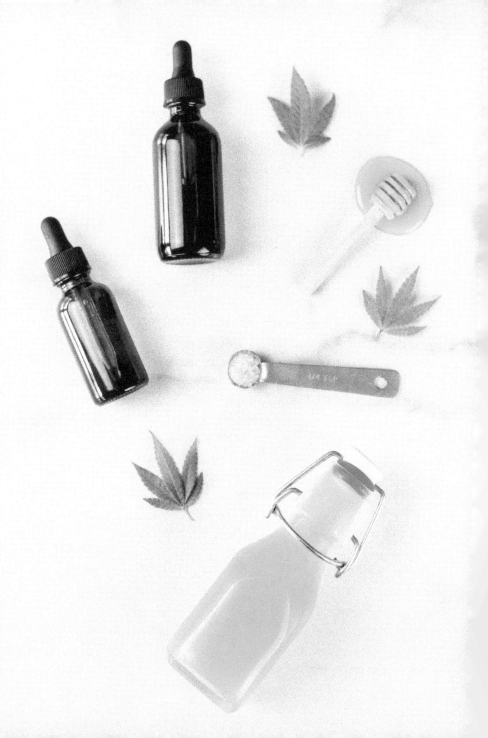

ISOLATES

Using an odorless and flavorless CBD isolate in a beverage is a fast and potent way to integrate CBD into your regimen. Available in a powder form or as a water-soluble nano-emulsified liquid concentrate, CBD isolate products are made from "isolated" CBD, where the CBD compound is extracted and separated from the rest of the plant. This means that all the other healing phytocannabinoids, terpenes, waxes, and oils are removed, leaving you with up to 99+ percent pure CBD. Be aware that most CBD isolate powder is not water soluble. If added to a beverage without infusing it into the drink properly, isolate powder will float on the top, which isn't appealing! To integrate isolate powder into the beverage properly, melt your desired amount into a liquid between 140°F and 150°F (60°C and 66°C). However, if you're creating smoothies or other blended drinks, heating doesn't matter as much. Just be sure to use a scale to measure your desired dose before putting the isolate into the blender.

If you use this method, be aware that isolates are typically not the most effective products to use because you're missing out on the entourage effect (page 10), and all the other beneficial phytocannabinoids, terpenes, flavonoids, waxes, and oils that contribute to cannabis's therapeutic properties.

PROFESSIONALLY MADE BAR PANTRY ITEMS

If you're not into making infused bar pantry items, there are now a variety of professionally made products you can purchase to assist in crafting cannabis-infused drinks. Similar to premade tinctures, these items are great options because they allow you to dose precisely. Look for infused honey, apple cider vinegar, cold brew coffee, infused tea sachets, cannabis-infused bitters and more. Flip to Resources on page 170 to see a selection of my favorite commercially made bar pantry items that are available now.

PITFALLS TO AVOID

After years of experimenting with cannabis-infused foods and drinks (and after making plenty of mistakes on my own), here are pitfalls to avoid when mixing cannabis into drinks.

USING TOP-SHELF PRODUCTS TO INFUSE DRINKS

Commercially made CBD and THC products can be very expensive, especially tinctures. If you have top-shelf items at home, consider setting them aside and looking for a less expensive (but still safe, clean, and lab-tested) option. Creating infusions at home using dry cannabis flower will also help you cut down on costs, plus you can make the infusion recipes in bulk. Just be sure that you're using clean, pesticide-free, flower sourced from a licensed dispensary or trusted farmer, or better yet, if you can, try to grow your own!

OVERHEATING PHYTOCANNABINOIDS AND TERPENES

When creating infusions at home, it's easy to get distracted and accidentally over-heat your cannabis flower during decarboxylation or the infusion process. High heat is extremely damaging to both phytocannabinoids and terpenes, so be sure to keep a constant eye on cooking temperatures, and when combined with a liquid, never let your cannabis or hemp flower boil. While using the stovetop is probably the most common method to creating infusions, sous vide is the most precise method because it keeps a constant temperature that helps preserve phytocanna-binoid and terpene profiles.

UNDERESTIMATING THE IMPORTANCE OF DOSING

While there is no universal standard for how much CBD or THC should be com-bined into a drink, it's best to start low and go slow. This is especially important if you're working with THC-infused ingredients. One of the most common mistakes is accidentally overserving yourself or a guest. If you're creating homemade infusions, always do the math to estimate the final cannabinoid percentages in each serving based on the specific batch of flower you use.

INTEGRATING CBD OR THC INTO DRINKS PROPERLY

To create a fantastic cannabis-infused drink, make sure to integrate the CBD or THC into your drink properly. Remember, the art of cannabis mixology is so much more complex than just adding tincture drops to your drink! Turn to page 74 to explore some recommended integration strategies.

MIXING CANNABIS AND ALCOHOL

While CBD does not have the same intoxicating effects as THC, the interactions between cannabidiol and alcohol have not been thoroughly researched. Some studies are showing that consuming both together doesn't seem to have any immediate adverse side effects, but always follow the golden rule, "start low go slow."

It's also been noted that alcohol may negate the effects of CBD due to the ways these substances interact when consumed together. If you're looking to get the most medicinal benefits from cannabis-infused drinks, I recommend sticking to zero-proof options including juices, smoothies, shakes, and other alcohol-free beverages. Do not mix with medications.

If you're making THC-infused cocktails, take extra precautions. I recommend staying below 5 milligrams of THC per drink or between 1 and 2.5 milligrams of THC for beginners. If you're mixing with high-proof alcohol or enjoying a drink that contains a few different spirits or liquors, drink only one drink max and stick to a microdose of THC. Do not overdo it.

Regardless of whether you're working with CBD or THC, pay close attention to how your body reacts after consuming a cannabis cocktail. Be patient. Avoid drinking multiple infused drinks in a row, even if you don't feel anything right away. Also, drink plenty of water to keep your body hydrated. And above all, do not drive or operate machinery after consuming cannabis-infused cocktails. Be smart and stay safe!

EXPLORING HOPS AND CANNABIS
+ HOW TO MAKE HOP TEA

featuring Jeremy Marshall, brewmaster for
Lagunitas Brewing Company & Hi-Fi Hops

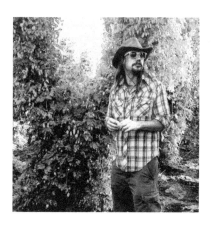

Jeremy Marshall is the brewmaster, or in his words, "Brewmonster," for
Lagunitas Brewing Company based in Sonoma County, California. As an
internationally known beer and dry-hopping expert, Jeremy has worked
closely with several of the top hop breeders and processors, contributing to
the development of several new hop varieties and hop-processing technologies
throughout his career. As an industry leader, he's guided Lagunitas's brews
since its early production days and has played a critical role in developing a
lineup of three unique CBD- and/or THC-infused beverages in partnership with
CannaCraft, aptly named Hi-Fi Hops. Follow Jeremy's latest beer creations
@lagunitasbeer and his latest cannabis-infused drinks @hifihops or visit
www.hifihops.com.

JEREMY MARSHALL: "I've always held a deep passion for *Cannabis sativa* and *Humulus lupulus*, the unpollinated female inflorescences commonly referred to as hops, which are used to both bitter and flavor all the world's beer. I especially like the intensely aromatic nature of IPAs, which are *dry-hopped,* the practice of adding hops to finished beer to allow the alcohol and water in fermented beer to extract the terpene-rich portion of the resinous glands of hops.

We should stop right there and make sure you're not thrown off by the rather trendy buzzword "terpene." If you're brand new to this term, the word gets its roots from turpentine, which is an old-school solvent made from pine sap. However, terpenes are almost like the pheromones of plants, often intensely aromatic and designed by plants as a messaging system, either to attract desirable things such as a pollinator or to ward off undesirable things, such as a predator.

Is there a cannabis strain that really does it for you because of the way it smells? For me, it's Jack Herer. If you also have a favorite aromatic strain, it's the terpene profile that you have to thank for that. As we often say, "the nose knows." There is some powerful truth to this. Terpenes are not only important for the overall psychopharmacological potential of cannabis and other botanical plants (and participants in the entourage effect), but the sense of smell is humankind's most primal sense. Smell bypasses the frontal cortex, or thinking brain, and goes straight into the animal brain, or limbic system, designed for pleasure, memory, and fight or flight. Ever had a smell suddenly trigger a memory, either good or bad? The smell of certain wooden antiques has the power to instantly take me right back to my grandparents' house thirty years ago! Perhaps there is something similar for you? Now let's get back to hops.

One does not have to like beer to appreciate hops, although many individuals are quick to point out that certain hop varietals "stink like weed," and beers designed by cannabis enthusiast brewers are often described as also smelling like cannabis. Hops grow around the world and the Germans perfected their use in beer. However, the British first used hops for dry hopping a pale ale that would then become known later as the "India Pale Ale" or IPA.

If we go back to about 26 or 27 million years ago into the two plants' evolutions well before humans, there was only a plant more closely resembling *Cannabis sativa*. As conditions on our lovely planet Earth evolved, cannabis tended toward the drier savannah habitats whereas *Humulus* is thought to have evolved and split off to chase the water-rich creek beds and riparian zones. Ask any hop farmer about how much water hops need and they will tell you all about it! The special part of the relationship is the terpene factory analogs of each plant: the trichome of cannabis and the lupulin gland of hops, which contain all the terpenes and all the brewing and/or medicinal value of the respective plants. Native Americans knew all about the medicinal properties of hops. They would make sedative teas to stimulate dream production and even stuff the ripe hop cones into pillows to sleep upon for a good night's rest.

If you'd like to try making hop tea yourself, I recommend starting with a pinch of fresh hops (both whole cones or pellets work) from your local brewpub or brewer, or a small 1-ounce (28-g) pack available online. Get fresh hops because the oils of old hops oxidize and smell quite a bit like cheese or hitchhiker's feet! Fresh hops should smell zesty with hints of pine, citrus, flowers, or slight skunk, depending on the variety. Boiling the hops or steeping them in hot water will create a rich, herbal bitterness. Shorter steep times and/or colder temperatures will promote the extraction of the terpenes. Terpenes are very heat sensitive and volatile, so delicate portions are best extracted at lower temperatures all the way down to 50°F (10°C).

Hops are similar to cannabis, but are more rich in myrcene (zesty, spicy, acrid, earthy), humulene (woody), beta-caryophyllene (peppery), linalool (floral), geraniol (geraniums, floral), pinene (pine sap), citronellol (citrus), and hundreds of other terpenes. Like cannabis, these terpenes serve as the romantic mystique separating the value and application of one varietal over another.

Developing Hi-Fi Hops is unique because it tastes like beer, yet it contains no alcohol or calories. It gets its terpene expression from hops while getting its medicinal value from cannabis. It was very much the accidental fruit of two groups of cool folks just hanging out. The intent was to ultimately seek a reunion of two ancient plants!"

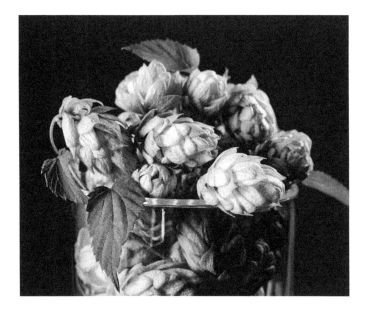

A GUIDE TO GLASSWARE

In the beverage world, choosing the correct glassware to serve your drinks in is incredibly important. It complements the drink's presentation and can enhance a beverage's characteristics. For example, think of the wine glass. There are specific glasses to be used for different categories of wine because the shape of the glass helps enhance the aromatic characteristics, which helps us interpret the wine's flavor profile.

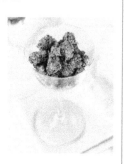

In addition to the many wine glasses and stemware that exist, there's also a wide variety of other glasses specifically designed for beer, cocktails, and nonalcoholic drinks such as coffee. Consider this your official glassware cheat sheet you can use as we explore cannabis drinks on a deeper level.

Classic Mug: Best for hot drinks, the classic mug is most often used for hot coffee or tea drinks.

Cocktail Coffee Glass: A clear and tall glass mug with a base and handle, most often used for drinks like the hot toddy and Irish coffee.

Collins Glass/Highball Glass: Tall and skinny, Collins glasses are usually a bit larger than the highball glass, but both are used for drinks that have ice in them and most often contain gin (Tom Collins), vodka (vodka soda), and sometimes whiskey (whiskey and gingers). Bloody Marys and tiki drinks also work well with these glasses, accommodating 8 to 12 ounces (240 to 360 ml) of liquid.

Copper Mug: Typically used for the Moscow mule or its variations, copper mugs are fantastic temperature conductors, either keeping your drink extra cold or extra hot.

Coupe Glass: Stylish and seductive, the coupe glass is often used for Champagne and sparkling wines or for drinks that are shaken or stirred with ice and served chilled, without ice. The coupe glass is a great alternative to the classic martini glass because it's not as likely to spill over.

Flute: Stemware most often used to serve sparkling wines, but also used for serving sparkling cocktails and sparkling spirit-free mixed drinks. Quick fact: In the wine industry, some Champagne producers are moving away from serving their sparklers in this style of glass because it's difficult to evaluate the aromas and flavors of the wine given the small circumference of the flute.

Martini Glass: Classically designed in a "V" shape, martini glasses are used for "straight up" drinks containing no ice. This glass can fit up to 5 ounces (150 ml) of liquid, but it's not the easiest glass to drink out of because it tends to spill over.

Nick & Nora Glass: As a trendy glass used in most high-end cocktail bars for "straight up" drinks, this glass is more bell-shaped than the coupe but smaller than the typical wine glass.

Old-Fashioned Glass: Also called a "rocks glass," this glass is used to showcase fine spirits or a spirit on the rocks. Typically holding up to eight ounces (240 ml), this glass is usually a bit heavier at the bottom and can accommodate either one big ice chunk or a handful of smaller ice cubes.

Pint Glass: The most common 16-ounce (480-ml) glass used to serve beer or cider. Fun fact! Similar to how there's a variety of styles of glasses to serve wine in, there are more than twenty styles of beer glasses that enhance the aromas and flavors of your favorite brews.

Shot Glass: Best for a quick 1 to 2 ounce (30 to 60 ml) shooter, the shot glass is used for spirits, mixed drinks, or healthy nonalcoholic fresh-pressed juice elixirs.

Wine Glass: Mostly used for wine and sometimes cocktails, such as the Aperol spritz, the wine glass is one the most diverse and specialized categories of glassware, ranging in a selection of different styles and shapes. Most often you'll encounter the traditional red wine glass, white wine glass, Bordeaux glass (used for Bordeaux varieties such as Cabernet Sauvignon, Merlot, Malbec), Burgundy glass (used for Pinot Noir and Italian Barolo and Barbaresco), White Burgundy glass, sparkling wine glass, fortified wine glass, and the universal all-purpose wine glass.

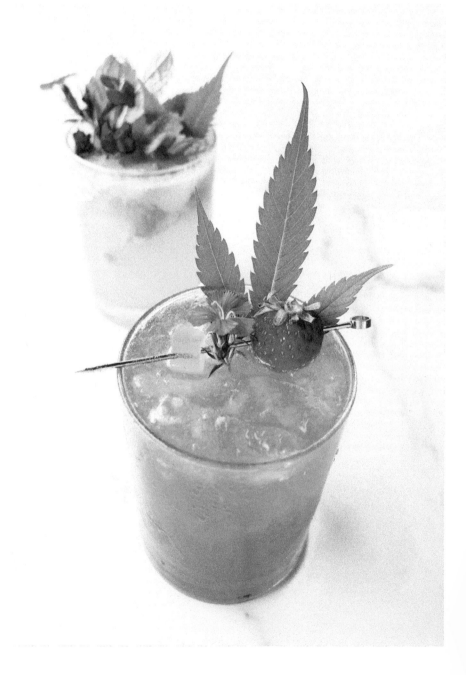

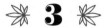

MASTERING INFUSIONS

To create the best cannabis-infused drinks at home, one of the most essential steps is learning how to create an infusion using cannabis flower. If you're new to infusions, it's a process of extracting organic compounds, such as CBD and THC, from cannabis by combining it with a solvent such as alcohol, oil, butter, or other fat-based and alcohol-based liquids. The goal when creating an infusion is to create a substance, such as cannabis-infused simple syrup, that can be integrated into a drink seamlessly.

Some of the most common methods for creating a heated infusion include stovetop, sous vide, slow cooker, or an infusion device. For this book, you'll mostly use the stovetop method for infusion. This fast and efficient infusion technique is fairly easy, plus you'll most likely already own the equipment that's called for. The biggest challenge with the stovetop technique is maintaining a consistent heating temperature when cooking. If you're looking for the most precise method and are willing to invest in a new tool, using a sous vide machine or infusion device (see Resources on page 170) is a terrific way to make elevated elixirs at home, especially if you're trying to preserve terpene profiles.

For alcohol-based infusions such as Infused Bitters (pages 66, 81), you'll use a different technique for infusion that doesn't require heat. All you'll need are some Mason jars and a dark pantry or freezer to store your infusion in.

Are you ready to create your very own cannabis bar pantry? Let's get started.

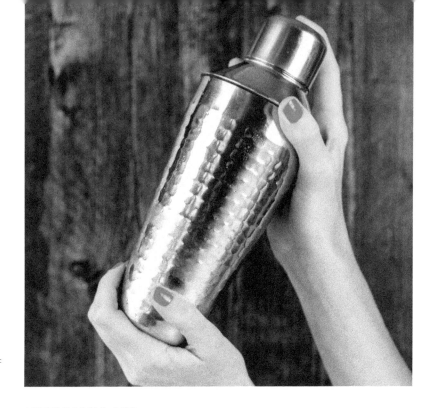

INFUSIONS 101

The first step to creating a drink infusion is deciding whether to use a fat-based or alcohol-based liquid for extracting CBD and THC. Whether you're using milk or spiced rum, before you make your first infusion, there are a few things you should be familiar with in each category. Let's explore these techniques in greater detail.

ALCOHOL-BASED INFUSIONS

Using alcohol to make a cannabis infusion is a common method that's been practiced for centuries. As the technique used to create alcohol-based cannabis tinctures, using grain alcohol, or ethanol, can easily extract phytocannabinoids, making this a dependable method when crafting infusions at home.

During the nineteenth and twentieth centuries, cannabis tinctures were widely used as a medicine, first appearing in the *United States Pharmacopoeia* in the 1850s. Unfortunately, due to the onset of cannabis prohibition in the United

States beginning in the 1930s, cannabis was later removed from the *United States Pharmacopoeia* in 1942. But, as we've seen today, alcohol-based cannabis tinctures have made a comeback and are a reliable way to consume the plant and receive its healing benefits. Plus, alcohol-based tinctures blend into drinks harmoniously without leaving behind unattractive oil residue.

Because of the high-yielding potency of alcohol extractions, only a small serving is needed when infusing a drink. Here are two methods you can use when creating alcohol-based infusions at home.

Non-Heated Alcohol Infusions

If you're planning on making an infusion using alcohol, keeping the alcohol at either room temperature or storing it in the freezer during the extraction process is the safest route; however, non-heated infusions take a long time to create. It might take several weeks to complete a recipe, but you do not need to add heat, which limits safety risks for at-home infusions.

To prepare, simply combine your choice of alcohol with decarboxylated cannabis flower in a sterilized Mason jar and store in a dark pantry or cabinet for 15 to 30 days, or in the freezer for up to 15 days. Agitate the mixture from time to time to help with the extraction process. Once the desired aromatics and flavor are achieved, strain the liquid through cheesecloth placed in a fine-mesh strainer to remove the sediment and store in an amber-colored tincture bottle or airtight swing bottle. If you're creating infused bitters, you can simply add the different fruits, herbs, spices, and botanical ingredients into a sterilized Mason jar and follow this same process. Remember that high-proof grain alcohol such as Everclear will yield the most potent infusions. Flip to page 80 for an alcohol-based infusion recipe using this technique.

Heated Alcohol Infusions

Heating alcohol can increase the efficiency of the extraction process and takes a shorter amount of time to complete. You must take extra precautions if you're planning to use this method at home: Alcohol is extremely flammable and has a low boiling point. Never use a gas stove when heating alcohol. Keep a close watch on cooking temperatures, heating the infusion well below 170°F (77°C) as alcohol flames at this point.

If you're thinking about making this type of infusion at home, I highly recommend using the sous vide method, especially if you'd like to make more precise, consistent infusions and you need the final product within two hours. You can also add various herbs, fruits, and spices to create different aromatic elements that enhance your drinks. Flip to page 79 for an infused alcohol tincture recipe using the sous vide method.

Fat-Washing

Fat-washing is an infusion technique you can use that relies on the extraction that occurs between fat flavor molecules and ethanol. This process has been known to make spirits a bit more smooth and creamy, or make cheaper spirits more pleasurable to consume. Because phytocannabinoids such as CBD and THC bind to both fat-based and alcohol-based solutions, the compounds extracted are infused into the spirit you're working with.

Ethanol-based solutions, such as gin, vodka, and rum, are best for this method because they can extract and dissolve different fats, leaving behind delicious fat flavors that have been combined with the alcohol base (think of buttered rum or bacon-flavored vodka).

To try this at home, start with a simple recipe such as cannabis-infused coconut rum. Simply combine 4 to 8 ounces (120 to 240 ml) of liquified cannabis-infused coconut oil with 750 milliliters of rum of your choice in a large sterilized Mason jar. Shake vigorously for a couple of minutes, then set the mixture in the freezer to chill overnight. The next morning, remove the liquid by poking a hole in the hardened fat that has risen to the top and strain before serving.

FAT-BASED INFUSIONS

Both CBD and THC are extremely drawn to fats, making them fat-soluble, lipophilic compounds. Because of their ability to bind with lipids and fats, you'll often come across CBD and THC products that have been combined with an oil. While oils can be tricky ingredients to work with when mixing with other liquids, there are a few occasions when you'll use them, particularly MCT oil. You can also create infusions using other fat-based liquids to combine with your cannabis flower including high-fat whole dairy milk, soymilk, and coconut milk. These are all fantastic options because of their high-fat content. Flip to page 104 for a fat-based tincture infusion recipe.

OTHER TECHNIQUES

Every now and then you might come across a drink recipe that does not contain alcohol or a fat-based liquid. If this is the case, don't fret! You can still create a potent infusion by adding food-grade vegetable glycerin or lecithin during the infusion process to help absorb phytocannabinoids. Food-grade vegetable glycerin is particularly useful if you're making infused simple syrup. It's also been known to accelerate the uptake of CBD and THC in your digestive system, which will help you feel effects more quickly. On the other hand, lecithin is a fat that can be found in many foods, including sunflowers, soybeans, and egg yolks. I've noticed that liquid sunflower lecithin typically works best for drink infusions or when combined with honey because it keeps ingredients from separating, in this case CBD or THC. For the recipes found in this book, using 1 to 2 tablespoons (15 to 30 ml) of glycerin or 1 to 2 teaspoons of liquid lecithin is recommended when creating a mixture that does not call for alcohol or a fat-based liquid. Head to your local health food store to find a reliable product.

DECARBOXYLATION

If you're looking to get the most out of your infusions and to create a more potent product, you must first decarboxylate your dry cannabis flower before integrating it into an infusion recipe. If you're new to decarboxylation, it is a heating process that triggers the chemical reaction that releases the carboxylic acids from CBD and THC to activate cannabis. In other words, the CBDA (the acidic precursor of CBD) and THCA (the nonintoxicating acidic precursor of THC) that's found in raw or dried cannabis flower is converted to CBD and THC when exposed to heat.

As you might have discovered, there are many decarboxylation methods you can use where activation is achieved by exposing dry cannabis to heat between 240°F to 295°F (115°C TO 146°C) for 20 to 60 minutes. If you're heating at higher temperatures, remember to decarboxylate for a shorter period of time. If you're heating at lower temperatures, heat for a longer period of time. Above all, do not exceed 300°F (150°C)—this will overheat your cannabis. Overheating can greatly degrade the important cannabinoids and terpenes that you're trying to preserve!

For the recipes in this book, I recommend using a decarboxylation technique known as the "oven method." To try this at home, preheat your oven to 275°F (140°C , or gas mark 1). As your oven is heating, line a baking sheet with aluminum foil or parchment paper. Begin to break up the dry flower into pea-size pieces with your fingers or scissors and spread the cannabis evenly onto your baking sheet. Once the oven is heated thoroughly, simply put the baking sheet in the oven and bake for 20 minutes. Remove from the heat and follow your recipe as noted.

NOTE: If you're using the oven method for decarboxylation, be aware that your house will fill up with very potent cannabis aromas when it is heated. If you're someone with a strict landlord or inquisitive neighbors, this method might not be your best option. Instead, try using a more discreet decarboxylation device such as the Ardent Nova, Ardent FX, or LEVO II. While decarboxylation is typically recommended, it's important to note that some chefs and mixologists prefer not to decarboxylate before cooking to help preserve terpene profiles. One of the best methods to use is the sous vide method, infusing the cannabis flower directly into your infusion base (i.e., alcohol, milk, butter, or olive oil) without preheating. It's up to you to determine what potency and flavor profile works best with the recipe you're creating, so keep these techniques in mind while crafting infusions.

DECARBOXYLATION AND COOKING TEMPERATURE GUIDE

As you cook with flower and other cannabis products, keeping a close eye on cooking temperatures is crucial. Here's a helpful decarboxylation and cooking temperature guide that will assist you as you explore infusions further.

ACTIVATION TEMPERATURES FOR DECARBOXYLATION

PHYTOCANNABINOIDS	°F	°C
THCA*	240–275	115–135
CBDA**	240–295	115– 146

*Converts from THCA to THC if you heat between 240°F and 275°F (115°C and 135°C) for 20 minutes to 1 hour

**Converts from CBDA to CBD if you heat between 240°F and 295°F (115°C and 146°C) for 20 minutes to 1 hour

BOILING POINTS

Stay below these temperatures to avoid the degradation of these important compounds:

PHYTOCANNABINOIDS	°F	°C
CBG	248	120
THC	314	157
CBD	320–356	160–180
CBDv	356	180
CBN	365	185
THCv	428	220
CBC	428	220

TERPENES	°F	°C
Humulene	252	122
Nerolidol	252	122
Beta-caryophyllene	266	130
Pinene	311	155
Myrcene	334	168
Limonene	349	176
Terpinolene	366	186
Linalool	388	198

CREATING YOUR INFUSED BAR PANTRY

Crafting cannabis drinks is easy once you have the right ingredients to mix. By creating an infused "bar pantry," you'll be able to quickly infuse several recipes using a few essential items. In the coming pages, you'll learn how to craft all these elixirs.

ALCOHOL-BASED TINCTURES

Having an alcohol-based tincture on hand is recommended. Rather than using a CBD or THC oil tincture, alcohol plays nicely with the other drink ingredients, infusing just about any beverage without separating out. See pages 79 to 80 for an infused alcohol tincture recipe.

INFUSED BITTERS

If you're looking to create delicious infused cocktails, having an array of cannabis bitters on hand is a must. If you're new to bitters, they are a flavoring agent used to blend drink flavors, most often made from different botanicals including fruits, flowers, spices, bark, roots, and other natural ingredients mixed with alcohol and a touch of water. Bitters are used in many classic cocktails and are celebrated by professional mixologists who often craft their own bitters to enhance a number of creations. Bitters can also add unique aromatics to a drink, making them an incredibly complex addition.

There are two types of bitters you should know: aromatic bitters and potable bitters. Aromatic bitters can be infused with just about any plant-based ingredient and are used by adding a few drops to a drink recipe. These bitters can help balance overly sweet drinks and add depth to beverages by adding more sophisticated aroma and flavor profiles for our palate to explore. Angostura and Peychaud's aromatic bitters are probably the two most well-known examples that represent this category.

Potable bitters (i.e., bitter liqueurs or amaros such as Campari and Fernet-Branca), are liqueurs infused with different botanicals, herbs, roots, spices, fruits, etc., and are drinkable on their own. Potable bitters tend to be lower in alcohol than aromatic bitters and can be sweeter on the palate, making them a great digestif.

For this book, you'll focus on creating aromatic cannabis-infused bitters using a combination of decarboxylated flower, alcohol, bittering agents (e.g., horehound, cinchona bark, wild cherry bark, orris root, gentian root, etc.) and flavoring agents (e.g., herbs, spices, fruits, fruit peels, etc.) mixed with a spirit containing at least 45 percent alcohol to help extract phytocannabinoids and essential oils. When these ingredients are combined, your infused bitters can microdose any drink with just a few dashes. Flip to page 81 for two infused bitters recipes.

INFUSED SHRUBS

Different from bitters, shrubs are classified as concentrated syrups that are created by combining vinegar, fresh fruit, sugar, spice, water, and sometimes alcohol. Sweet yet tart, these vinegar-based syrups are incredibly refreshing and can be easily combined with mixers to create craft drinks. Shrubs are a trendy, complex addition to a number of beverages, but are also flavorful enough to enjoy with just sparkling water or club soda because of all the mouthwatering seasonal fruits and vegetables that can be used in shrub recipes.

While there are several methods for creating shrubs at home, I prefer using the cold process method rather than heating the ingredients, although some shrubs do require heat (see page 137). The cold process method extracts the pure, fresh flavors of the fruit, delivering bright aromas and flavors that best express the essence of your ingredients. Even though the hot process is faster, the fruit used in your recipe can often take on a jammy, cooked flavor, which isn't as great as the outcome when cold processing.

So, how do you infuse a shrub with cannabis? The recipes found throughout this book call for an infused alcohol tincture that you can artfully blend into the shrub ingredients upon making it. Flip to pages 79 to 80 for three infused shrub recipes.

INFUSED HONEY

Cannabis-infused honey is an incredibly versatile ingredient because it mixes seamlessly into several beverages including hot tea, smoothies, and other hot drinks. CBD and THC honey is also easy to make at home, requiring only a few simple ingredients: organic honey and your preferred hemp or cannabis oil.

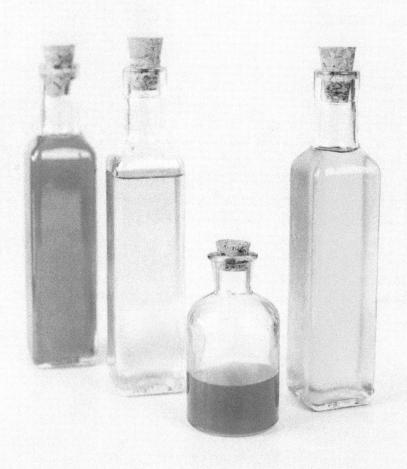

On its own, honey provides many therapeutic benefits as it's full of antioxidants. It also provides our bodies with beneficial enzymes and nutrients, and acts as a substitute for artificial sweeteners. When combined with cannabis, honey is the optimal partner to transport the many health-giving benefits that help maintain homeostasis. Because it's one of the most easily digested forms of carbohydrates, it's a prime vehicle to deliver herbal medicine, in this case CBD or THC, into the body.

To learn more about the magic of infused honey and how you can incorporate it into your drink regimen, flip to page 71 and meet the founders of Potli.

INFUSED SIMPLE SYRUP

Another important staple in your infused bar pantry is creating infused simple syrup. A simple syrup most often consists of a sugar base, such as granulated sugar, honey, or agave nectar mixed with water over heat. There are many ways you can spice them up. To make your simple syrup recipes more complex, you can add herbs, fruits, nuts, and spices during the heating process including cinnamon, cardamom, lemon, ginger, and lavender. Infused simple syrup adds sweetness to your drinks and can also help balance acidity and bitterness, while rounding out harsher alcohol characteristics when making cocktails.

When infusing a simple syrup with cannabis or hemp flower, the primary ingredients you'll be working with do not include an alcohol-based or fat-based liquid. So, how do you capture the CBD or THC? To extract the cannabinoids and create a successful infusion, you'll want to add 1 tablespoon (15 ml) of food-grade vegetable glycerin, which will act as your fat base. For a seasonal selection of infused simple syrups, flip to page 90.

INFUSED SOUR MIX

If you're a fan of margaritas or pisco sours, having a homemade infused sour mix on hand is a helpful bar essential that can quickly add tangy, citrus flavors to a drink recipe. While premade sour mixes can taste awful and sometimes toxic, creating your own recipe at home using fresh lemon and lime juices is an enjoyable tasting experience. Combining infused rich simple syrup with citrus juices, this easy-to-make recipe can also be added to zesty vinaigrettes to liven up a salad. Flip to page 93 for an infused sour mix recipe.

HOW TO INCREASE THE POTENCY OF DIY INFUSIONS

When creating DIY infusions at home, keep in mind that the recipes called for in this chapter have been crafted to accommodate low to medium CBD and THC dosing. If you're someone who prefers a more potent infusion, there are a few techniques that you can use to increase the target dose to best accommodate your needs.

TECHNIQUE 1: Choose a strain with a high potency to craft your infusions. For example, if you're looking for a stronger dose of THC, choose a strain that's THC-rich ranging between 15 to 25 percent or more THC by dry weight. The more CBD or THC that your flower contains, the stronger your infusion will be.

TECHNIQUE 2: Increase the amount of decarboxylated flower that's called for in each infusion recipe. While this technique isn't the most ideal, if you choose to do so, you can increase the potency of the infusion by adding more decarboxylated flower. Keep in mind, this technique might lead to a stronger cannabis flavor.

TECHNIQUE 3: For those who require a high dose, you can also simply use a commercially made high-potency tincture to infuse the drinks versus making an infusion. Just remember to use precautions and sample the product to gauge potency before mixing it into a drink.

WHAT'S NOT RECOMMENDED: Once you've crafted the infusions and you're ready to start mixing them into the drink recipes found in chapters 4 and 5, do not add more than what's called for in each recipe to increase the target dose. This is especially important for ingredients, such as simple syrup, that can drastically change the flavor profile of the drink if too much is added. For best results, stick to techniques 1, 2, or 3 to increase the potency of your infusions or drinks.

THE POWERS OF CBD HONEY AND HOW TO MIX IT INTO DRINKS

featuring Felicity Chen and Christine Yi, founders of Potli

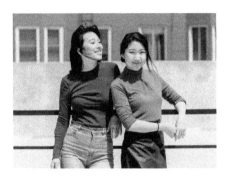

The Potli story begins with founders Felicity Chen and Christine Yi's cannabis-infused honey, which is harvested from their own hives in the San Francisco Bay Area. As their flagship product, Potli's honey was first created to help aid Felicity's mother's asthma. With her in mind, this dynamic duo set out to craft a product that consumers can trust, where quality and dosage is undoubtedly clear and apparent. Later expanding into a full line of cannabis- and hemp-infused pantry items, the Potli team offers infused honey, olive oil, chili oil, and sriracha. Follow Felicity, Christine, and Potli @getpotli or visit www.potlishop.com.

FELICITY CHEN & CHRISTINE YI: "Long before we started a business together, Christine and I met in New England as randomly paired roommates our freshman year of college. During that first semester away, I remember catching a terrible cold, the never-ending kind that makes you swear that you'll take full advantage of your health once you recover. As a proponent for holistic medicine, Christine took care of me by mixing teas with herbs or lemon and honey to soothe my throat, setting the tone for our friendship. Since then, the potential to soothe oneself or care for others using natural ingredients has been a primary motivation as we've created our cannabis-infused panty item line, Potli.

Our signature raw honey is a product that we hand-harvest in the San Francisco Bay Area, where my father first started beekeeping to make hyper-local honey for my mother's asthma. We were inspired to create Potli for her, and for people like her, who have so much to gain from the anti-inflammatory and pain-relieving properties of cannabis, yet would never feel comfortable smoking it.

In ancient Ayurvedic medicine, honey is considered yogavahi, or the most powerful vessel for herbal remedies, capable of penetrating the deepest layers of our bodies. At Potli, we combine it with cannabis to create a superfood that's antibacterial and high in antioxidants, a powerful anti-inflammatory agent that can help soothe the body. Cannabis and hemp-infused honey is nourishing and can even help fight allergies. It also provides an incredible depth of flavor with unique seasonal tasting notes that pair well with many different types of beverages.

To experience the powers of CBD-infused honey and to learn how to mix it into beverages, we've put together a recipe for you to experiment with. We love our CBD or THC infused honey in drinks ranging from cold-busting teas to anti-hangover cocktails. To get you started, here's our Relaxing Bedtime Elixir. We hope you enjoy!"

POTLI BEDTIME ELIXIR

Unwind and restore with this calming bedtime tea. This recipe helps promote muscle relaxation and hormone regulation to help you fall and stay asleep.

YIELD: **1** serving

TARGET DOSE: 10 mg CBD per tablespoon (using Potli honey) or 15 mg CBD per tablespoon (using Full-Spectrum Infused Honey, page 91).

EQUIPMENT
Small saucepan
Measuring spoons
Teacup or mug

INGREDIENTS
1½ cups (360 ml) unsweetened almond milk or milk of your choice

1 chamomile tea sachet or buds

2 slices fresh ginger to steep (or ½ teaspoon grated fresh ginger)

1 tablespoon (21 g) Potli Hemp-Infused Honey or 1 tablespoon (21g) DIY Full-Spectrum Infused Honey (page 91)

½ teaspoon ashwagandha powder

½ teaspoon reishi powder

¼ teaspoon rhodiola powder

Using a small saucepan, heat the unsweetened almond milk over low heat. Once the almond milk begins to simmer, remove from the heat and pour into a teacup. Steep the chamomile and ginger in the warmed almond milk. Add the infused honey, ashwagandha, reishi, and rhodiola. Stir together until blended well and enjoy warm.

NOTE: *Instead of chamomile, try steeping lavender buds for an aromatherapy experience or add coconut or MCT oil for a thicker, frothier tea.*

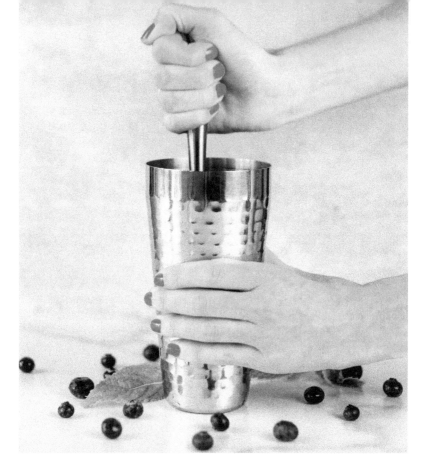

TECHNIQUES FOR INTEGRATING CBD OR THC OIL INTO DRINKS

When creating cannabis-infused drinks at home, one primary goal is making sure the CBD or THC that you're integrating into the beverage doesn't separate from the rest of the ingredients that you're working with. While creating your own cannabis-infused bar pantry items limits this risk, sometimes you'll be working with a commercially made CBD or THC oil to craft infused drinks. Combining oil with liquids can be extremely challenging, however, there are a few techniques you can use to create the most well-balanced drinks possible. Similar to cooking, these emulsification techniques allow you to combine unlikely ingredients to prevent separation. Here are a few common ways to integrate CBD or THC oils into your beverages.

BLENDING

If you're planning on making a cannabis-infused smoothie, shake, or cocktail, blending is a fantastic way to integrate infused ingredients into your drinks. By blending, the machine does the work for you, breaking apart the CBD or THC oil droplets so they mix into the other liquids and ingredients seamlessly.

MIXING AND STIRRING

Hand mixing via a whisk or stirring using a mixing glass and a bar spoon is another technique you can use to emulsify ingredients. While not as efficient as using a blender, if you thoroughly mix or stir the ingredients together, you can temporarily emulsify the oil drops into the drink. I've found it's best to mix or stir drinks for about 1 minute to properly combine.

MUDDLING

When using CBD or THC oil in a drink, another technique you can use is muddling. Muddling works best when you combine cannabis oil with different fruits or herbs, simple syrup or juice at the bottom of a glass, then apply pressure with a muddler to muddle/emulsify the ingredients. This technique also releases the flavors of the fresh ingredients that you're working with, allowing the muddled mixture to bind with your liquid ingredients more easily. If you use this technique in a shaker tin, be aware that you'll encounter some loss of cannabinoids after straining the liquids from the solids, but overall it's a good method for combining the ingredients.

SHAKING

Using a cocktail shaker tin to integrate CBD and THC is another technique you can use when crafting cannabis beverages at home. This works best for drinks that include fruit juices and citrus, plus other "cloudy" ingredients such as egg whites and dairy. Remember, the more you vigorously shake, the better the CBD or THC will mix into the other liquids. If you're using an oil, separation will occur over time, but you can easily re-emulsify by putting the drink back into your shaker tin and vigorously shaking once again.

    WARNING: Never put carbonated ingredients, such as club soda or sparkling water, into the shaker tin! If you do, it could explode and you'll have a big mess to clean up.

THE SCIENCE BEHIND THE BOOMING CANNABIS BEVERAGE CATEGORY

featuring Ben Larson & Dr. Harold Han of Vertosa

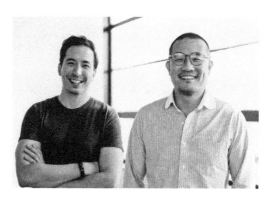

Nanoemulsion expert, Dr. Harold Han, and cannabis-industry investor and business adviser, Ben Larson, joined forces in 2018 to launch Vertosa, creators of industry-leading active ingredients for infused product makers. Their patent-pending nano- and microemulsions are carefully designed for the specific needs of each customer, with presuspended aqueous solutions that create incredibly homogeneous and stable products while maximizing bioavailability, clarity, and taste. Vertosa works closely with their lab partners and clients of all sizes throughout the manufacturing process to achieve the desired consumer experience and target potency, and to accelerate products to market. Learn more about Vertosa at vertosa.com or follow @vertosainc.

BEN LARSON & DR. HAROLD HAN: "Some of the strongest scientific innovation in cannabis is happening around beverages. Gone are the days of bitter, unstable, or dubiously effective infused cannabis drinks.

Consumers now have access to myriad beverages that provide low-dose, sessionable, and consistent experiences. Better yet, we're able to do so in great tasting, low-calorie form factors that don't require the addition of excessive amounts of sweetener.

The key to these new beverage formats is emulsion technology—disrupting the antagonistic relationship between oil and water. By breaking down cannabis oils into presuspended liquid nanoemulsions (droplets less than 100 nanometers in size) and microemulsions (typically ranging from 100 to 400 nanometers) we can now infuse everything from wine to beer to cold brew coffee with CBD and THC, among other cannabinoids and terpenes.

By creating custom solutions for each specific product, oil droplets are encapsulated and evenly dispersed into the beverage. The small hydrophilic (water-friendly) droplets allow the cannabinoids to absorb into the bloodstream faster, creating a quicker onset, while increasing the overall absorption. What does this all mean? We can more accurately create low-dose products that result in an easy-to-manage imbibing experience while lowering the potential for over-consumption.

At Vertosa, one of the reasons we've been able to infuse beverage brands ranging from House of Saka to Vita Coco, is that we don't settle for a one-size-fits-all mentality. Infusion solutions should be carefully tailored to fit the needs of each partner's intended experience, including taste, clarity, mouthfeel, stability, and compatibility. Thanks to scientific innovation, beverages are primed to make cannabis more accessible to, and more approachable for, a wider array of people than ever before. Limitless possibilities abound for the future of customized beverages."

INFUSION RECIPES

Now that you've learned about all the many ways to make cannabis drink infusions, it's time to put your skills to the test and create infused mixers, including bitters, shrubs, honey, simple syrup, and sour mix, by combining different ingredients primarily with dried cannabis flower.

For this book, I infused these recipes using a strain called Cannatonic, which measured at a total of 12 percent CBD and 3 percent THC before decarboxylation. These numbers will differ depending on the strain and source of the product you use, so be sure to calculate your own CBD/THC milligrams per serving before making your infusion (refer to page 33 for at-home dosage calculations).

Remember that the target dosage listed in each recipe can simply be a baseline for your infusions, but your final outcome will vary depending on the flower you use. When crafting infusions at home, always try to make an accurate estimate and sample each infusion with conservative tastings before serving to others to gauge the potency.

If you're not into making recipes using cannabis or hemp flower, or want to avoid THC altogether, you can easily craft these infusion recipes using a CBD isolate. Just keep in mind that you'll be missing out on the other healing phytocannabinoids, terpenes, flavonoids, and oils that contribute to the entourage effect (which improves CBD's efficacy).

*IMPORTANT: When crafting drink infusions, to avoid overly bitter flavors, I recommend removing the cannabis stems from the decarboxylated cannabis flower before it goes into your infusion recipe. While stem flavors are less noticeable in infusions such as Infused Bitters (page 81), if you're infusing something more delicate, such as milk, leave the stems out.

Now, on to the infusion recipes!

INFUSED ALCOHOL TINCTURE, TWO WAYS

For your first infusion, you'll want to create an infused alcohol tincture that can be mixed into just about any recipe. By combining high-proof alcohol with decarboxylated cannabis flower, you can easily extract important phytocannabinoids that will enhance your beverages. Whether you use the heated sous vide method for infusion or the unheated method (storing the mixture in the freezer during the infusion process), you can count on this tincture to be the most versatile item in your bar pantry. Plus, it's what you'll use to infuse shrub recipes found in this chapter!

SOUS VIDE METHOD

YIELD: about 6 ounces (180 ml)	**TARGET DOSE:** 2 mg CBD | < 1 mg THC per milliliter or 52 mg CBD | 13 mg THC per ounce (30 ml)

EQUIPMENT
Vacuum seal bags
Sous vide device
Cheesecloth
Fine-mesh strainer
8-ounce (240-ml) sterilized
    Mason jar, airtight swing
    bottle, or split between
    amber glass bottles with
    dropper cap

INGREDIENTS
1 cup (240 ml) Everclear
4.5 grams decarboxylated
    flower of your choice

Set your sous vide water bath to 140°F (60°C). Combine the Everclear with the decarboxylated flower and pour the mixture into a pouch using a vacuum seal bag. Double check the bag to make sure it's airtight! Sous vide the pouch for 2 hours, then remove from the heat. Let the pouch cool to room temperature before straining out the flower. For best results, place the cheesecloth in a fine-mesh strainer and strain into a jar. Store in a dark pantry for up to 1 year.

WARNING: *Never use a gas stove or open flame when working with alcohol-based infusions. Remember that Everclear is highly flammable and should never be heated at or above 170°F (77°C).*

NOTE

The sous vide method is recommended for heating and is a great technique to use because it provides precise temperature control. Remember that by using the sous vide technique, you're preventing any volatile aromas or vapor from escaping, which can actually amplify the flavors of your alcohol infusion.

FREEZER METHOD

If you prefer to avoid a heated method for infusion, you can still create this recipe by combining 4.5 grams decarboxylated flower with 1 cup (240 ml) Everclear in a 16-ounce (480-ml) Mason jar. Seal the jar tightly and place it in the freezer for 15 days. By freezing, you're preventing the strong herbaceous notes from flavoring the tincture, which leaves you with a cleaner-tasting product. Make sure to agitate the jar every day to help with the extraction process. After the 15 days are up, line a fine-mesh strainer with cheesecloth and filter out the solids from the infused alcohol. For optimal clarity, filter twice. Store in a dark pantry for up to 1 year.

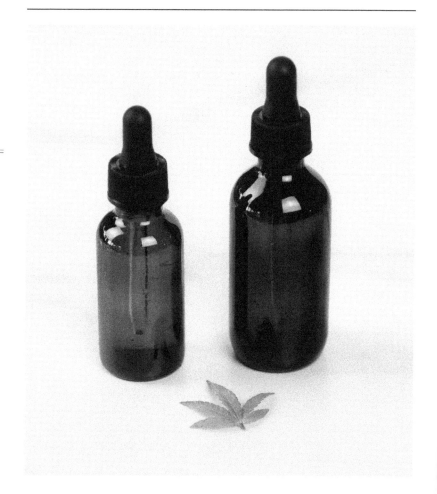

INFUSED BITTERS, TWO WAYS

Having a selection of cannabis bitters on hand is a fantastic way to microdose CBD and THC into a number of beverages, particularly craft cocktails. While there are a few different methods for creating bitters at home, a great place to start if you're a beginner is to experiment with the "combination method," meaning you combine the bittering and flavoring ingredients into one Mason jar for infusion. While this method isn't as precise as using the "tincture method" for combining flavors and aromas, it's convenient, easy, and requires much less time and prep. To support an array of complex beverages, here are two infused bitters recipes.

INFUSED CITRUS SPICE BITTERS

YIELD: about **16** ounces (480 ml)	**TARGET DOSE:** 2 mg CBD | < 1 mg THC per ¼ teaspoon or 2 dashes (12 to 16 drops)

EQUIPMENT
One 32-ounce (960-ml) sterilized Mason jar
Two 16-ounce (480-ml) sterilized Mason jars
One 8-ounce (240-ml) sterilized Mason jar
Cheesecloth
Fine-mesh strainer
Airtight swing bottle or amber bottle with a dropper cap

INGREDIENTS
10 grams decarboxylated flower of your choice
¼ cup (24 g) dried lemon peel
¼ cup (24 g) dried orange peel
5 cardamom pods, cracked
½ heaping teaspoon cinchona bark

1 cinnamon stick
1 (1-inch or 2.5-cm) piece fresh ginger, peeled and cut into thin slices
2 cups (480 ml) high-proof rye
¾ cup (180 ml) water
½ ounce (15 ml) non-infused rich simple syrup (optional)

Add the decarboxylated flower, citrus, cardamom, cinchona bark, cinnamon, and ginger to a 32-ounce (960-ml) Mason jar. Top with high-proof rye, seal, and shake vigorously. Steep this mixture for 15 days, stored in a dark pantry. Shake daily.

After the 15 days are up, separate the solids from the liquids through cheesecloth placed in a fine-mesh strainer set over a clean 16-ounce (480-ml) Mason jar. Reserve the solids. Seal the Mason jar filled with the citrus spice–infused alcohol and store it in a dark pantry until further use.

(continued)

Transfer the solids into a small saucepan along with the water. Cook over medium heat for about 6 minutes. Remove from the heat and let cool. Once the mixture reaches room temperature, transfer it to a clean 16-ounce (480-ml) Mason jar and steep for 3 days in the refrigerator, agitating daily.

Once the 3 days are up, separate the liquid from the solids through cheesecloth placed in a fine-mesh strainer set over a clean 8-ounce (240-ml) Mason jar, then discard the solids/sediment. Double filter if needed to help with clarity and add the rich simple syrup (if using) into the liquid. Shake to combine, then add this liquid mixture to the citrus spice–infused alcohol that you've already created.

Shake well, then let the bitters rest for a few more days, allowing the sediment to sink to the bottom of the Mason jar. Once the 2 or 3 days are up, carefully filter out the clean liquid that's resting on top through cheesecloth placed in a fine-mesh strainer set over a clean bowl. Leave the sediment behind, then discard. Store the infused bitters in an airtight swing bottle or separate into smaller amber bottles with a dropper cap. Keep at room temperature for up to 1 year, and store in a dark pantry for best results.

HOW TO DRY CITRUS PEELS

To prepare dried lemon or orange peels, preheat the oven to 200°F (93°C). Line a baking sheet with parchment paper and set aside. Peel the citrus into thin strips using a peeler. Remove just the yellow or orange part of the citrus—no pith. Spread the citrus across the baking sheet and place in the oven. Bake for 45 minutes to 1 hour, or until all the citrus strips are dried out and the ends curl up. Let rest for 2 to 3 hours before using.

INFUSED CELERY BITTERS

YIELD: about **16** ounces (480 ml)	**TARGET DOSE:** 2 mg CBD | < 1 mg THC per ¼ teaspoon or 2 dashes (12 to 16 drops)

EQUIPMENT

One 32-ounce (960-ml)
    sterilized Mason jar
Two 16-ounce (480-ml)
    sterilized Mason jars
One 8-ounce (240-ml)
    sterilized Mason jar
Fine-mesh strainer
Cheesecloth
Swing bottle or amber bottle
    with a dropper cap

INGREDIENTS

**10 grams decarboxylated
    flower of your choice**

**1 cup (100 g) finely chopped
    celery**

1 teaspoon celery seeds

**1 tablespoon (5 g) coriander
    seeds**

1 teaspoon fennel seeds

**¼ teaspoon fresh dill,
    chopped**

**4 fresh mint leaves, cut into
    thin strips**

**¼ heaping teaspoon gentian
    root**

**¼ heaping teaspoon
    horehound**

**2 cups (480 ml) Everclear or
    high-proof vodka**

¾ cup (180 ml) water

Add the decarboxylated flower, celery, celery seed, coriander seeds, fennel seeds, dill, mint, gentian root, and horehound into a 32-ounce (960-ml) Mason jar. Top with Everclear, seal, and shake vigorously. Steep this mixture for 15 days, stored in a dark pantry. Shake daily.

Separate the solids from the liquids through cheesecloth placed in a fine-mesh strainer set over a clean 16-ounce (480-ml) Mason jar. Reserve the solids. Seal the Mason jar and store it in a dark pantry until further use.

Next, transfer the solids into a small saucepan along with the water. Cook over medium heat for about 6 minutes. Remove from the heat and let cool. Once the mixture reaches room temperature, transfer it to a clean 16-ounce (480-ml) Mason jar and steep for 3 days in the refrigerator, agitating daily.

Once the 3 days are up, separate the liquid from the solids through cheesecloth placed in a fine-mesh strainer set over a clean 8-ounce (240-ml) Mason jar, then discard the solids/sediment. Double filter if needed to help with clarity, then add this liquid mixture to the celery-infused alcohol you've already created.

Shake well, then let the bitters rest for a few more days, allowing the sediment to sink to the bottom of the Mason jar. Once the 2 or 3 days are up, carefully filter out the clean liquid that's resting on top through cheesecloth placed in a fine-mesh strainer. Leave the sediment behind, then discard. Store the infused bitters in an airtight swing bottle or separate into smaller amber bottles with a dropper cap. Keep at room temperature for up to 1 year, and store in a dark pantry for best results.

MASTERING INFUSIONS

INFUSED SHRUBS,
THREE WAYS

When it comes to drinks, I highly recommend making shrubs. They are a fun and flavorful way to add CBD and THC into your beverages. Using a variety of fresh fruits combined with vinegar and sugar, shrubs add complexity, offering the perfect balance of sweet and sour flavors. These recipes blend some of the most delicious flavor combinations—ginger and peach, strawberry and lime, and grapefruit and rosemary—and they will take your cannabis drinks to a heightened level.

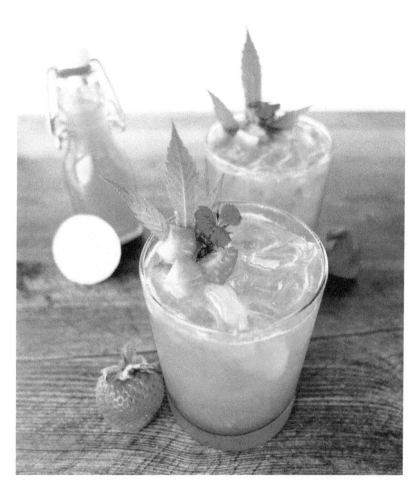

INFUSED GINGER PEACH SHRUB

YIELD: about 16 ounces (480 ml)	**TARGET DOSE:** 3 mg CBD | 1 mg THC per ounce (30 ml) using Infused Alcohol Tincture (page 79)

EQUIPMENT
Mixing bowls
Grater
Plastic wrap
Strainer
Whisk
Funnel
Airtight swing bottle

INGREDIENTS
2 cups (340 g) fresh ripe yellow peaches, pitted and cut into pieces
1 cup (200 g) sugar
1 (1½-inch or 3.5-cm) piece fresh ginger, peeled
1 cup (240 ml) champagne vinegar
1 ounce (30 ml) Infused Alcohol Tincture (page 79)

Combine the peaches and sugar in a small mixing bowl, then grate the fresh ginger into the bowl. Stir together until the sugar coats each piece, then use a fork to mash the peaches slightly. Cover the bowl with plastic wrap or a lid and store in the refrigerator overnight to macerate.

The next day, give the mixture a few good stirs, then use a strainer to separate the peach solids from the newly formed syrup over a mixing bowl. Set the solids aside.

In a mixing bowl, add the champagne vinegar and whisk. Using a clean bowl, pour the ginger peach syrup and vinegar blend over the fruit solids to collect any remaining sugar that might be leftover. Repeat this step a few times to get all the remaining sugar. Discard the solids.

Add the infused alcohol tincture to the mixing bowl with the other liquids. Whisk together, then funnel the shrub into an airtight swing bottle. Store in the refrigerator for 2 to 3 days before using. If stored properly, this shrub should stay fresh for several weeks. Shake well before serving.

NOTE For optimal results, source fresh and ripe yellow peaches rather than white peaches for brighter color and a more pronounced peach flavor.

INFUSED STRAWBERRY LIME SHRUB

YIELD: about 14 ounces (420 ml)	**TARGET DOSE:** 4 mg CBD	1 mg THC per ounce (30 ml) using Infused Alcohol Tincture (page 79)

EQUIPMENT

Zester
Mixing bowls
Mixing spoon
Plastic wrap
Strainer
Whisk
Funnel
Airtight swing bottle

INGREDIENTS

2 organic limes
1½ cups (255 g) strawberries, cut into quarters
½ cup (100 g) sugar
1 cup (240 ml) apple cider vinegar
1 ounce (30 ml) Infused Alcohol Tincture (page 79)

Zest the limes over a mixing bowl. Combine the lime zest with the strawberries and sugar. Stir together until the sugar coats the strawberries completely. Cover the bowl with plastic wrap and store in the refrigerator overnight to macerate.

The next day, give the mixture a good stir and use a strainer to separate the newly formed syrup from the berry solids over a mixing bowl. Set the solids aside. To the bowl containing the strawberry lime syrup, add the apple cider vinegar, then whisk together. Using a clean bowl, pour the syrup and vinegar blend over the solids to collect any remaining sugar that might be leftover. Repeat this step a few times to collect all the remaining sugar. Discard the solids.

Add the infused alcohol tincture to the mixing bowl with the other liquids. Whisk again, then funnel the shrub into an airtight swing bottle. Store in the refrigerator for an additional 2 to 3 days before using. If stored properly, this shrub should stay fresh for a couple of weeks. Shake well before serving.

CANNABIS DRINKS

INFUSED GRAPEFRUIT ROSEMARY SHRUB

YIELD: about **14** ounces (420 ml)	**TARGET DOSE:** 4 mg CBD | 1 mg THC per ounce (30 ml) using Infused Alcohol Tincture (page 79)

EQUIPMENT
Small mixing bowls
Muddler
Peeler
Plastic wrap
Fine-mesh strainer
Whisk
Funnel
Airtight swing bottle

INGREDIENTS
3 rosemary sprigs

¾ cup (180 ml) champagne vinegar

Zest of 2 organic ruby red grapefruits, peeled into strips

½ cup (100 g) sugar

1 ounce (30 ml) Infused Alcohol Tincture (page 79)

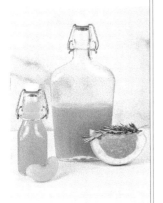

Begin by preparing the rosemary-infused vinegar. The day before you plan to serve your drinks, remove the rosemary leaves from the stems and place the leaves in a bowl, cover with champagne vinegar, slightly muddle, then place in the refrigerator overnight.

The next day, over a small mixing bowl, use a peeler to remove as much of the grapefruit peel as possible—no pith! Add the sugar, stir together, then muddle the ingredients. Cover the bowl with plastic wrap and let sit for 1½ hours. As the grapefruit sugar is resting, juice the grapefruits through a fine-mesh strainer over a mixing bowl to remove the pulp and set aside. Remove the rosemary vinegar from the refrigerator, then use a fine-mesh strainer to separate the solids from the liquids over the same mixing bowl that contains the grapefruit juice. Set aside.

After the 1½ hours are up, add the grapefruit juice and rosemary vinegar blend into the mixing bowl, covering the grapefruit sugar and sugared peels. Use a whisk to blend, then pour the mixture through a fine-mesh strainer into a clean mixing bowl to remove the peels and extra pulp. Using a clean bowl, pour the syrup and vinegar blend back over the grapefruit peels to collect any remaining sugar that might be leftover. Discard the solids.

Add the infused alcohol tincture and whisk again well. Using a funnel, transfer the shrub into an airtight swing bottle. Give it a couple of good shakes, then store in the refrigerator for 2 to 3 days before using. If stored properly, this shrub should stay fresh for several weeks.

SEASONAL INFUSED SIMPLE SYRUPS

To add a touch of sweetness to your cannabis-infused drinks, having a selection of cannabis-infused simple syrups on hand will enhance your recipes effortlessly. Celebrating terpene-inspired aromas and flavors, here are a few recipes to stock your bar pantry. As you work your way through this book, you will use a lot of rich simple syrup, so I adjusted the yield to account for this. For best results, store in the refrigerator and keep cool until serving.

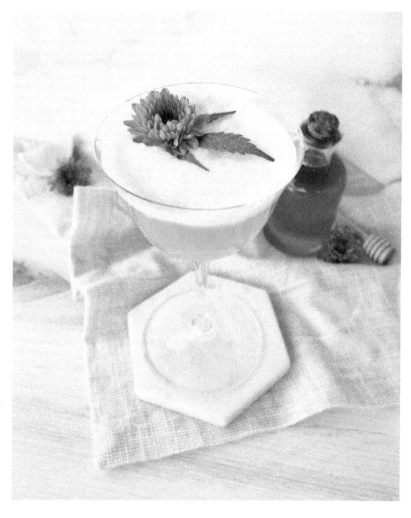

INFUSED RICH SIMPLE SYRUP

YIELD: about 28 ounces (840 ml)	**TARGET DOSE:** 15 mg CBD | 4 mg THC per ounce (30 ml) (using a flower infusion)

EQUIPMENT
Digital scale
Measuring cups
Measuring spoons
Small saucepan
Thermometer
One 32-ounce (960-ml)
    sterilized Mason jar
Cheesecloth
Fine-mesh strainer

INGREDIENTS
**5 grams decarboxylated
    flower of your choice**
**4 cups (800 g) granulated
    sugar**
2 cups (480 ml) water
**1 tablespoon (15 ml) food-
    grade vegetable glycerin**

Before making this recipe, remember that when preparing a rich simple syrup, it's sweeter than a normal simple syrup, so your sugar base should be a greater ratio than the water that's called for.

Weigh 5 grams of decarboxylated flower. Set aside.

Combine the sugar and water in a small saucepan. Bring to a soft boil, stirring until the sugar dissolves into the water. Reduce the heat to between 160°F to 180°F (71°C to 82°C) and add the decarboxylated cannabis.

Simmer over low heat for 50 minutes, stirring occasionally, scraping the sides of the pan to remove flower and sugar debris. Reduce the heat and add the vegetable glycerin—this will give the CBD (and THC) something to bind to. Continue to heat and stir for 10 minutes. Remove from the heat.

Pour the infused simple syrup into a 32-ounce (960-ml) Mason jar through cheesecloth placed in a fine-mesh strainer to separate the solids. Let cool and shake before serving.

Store in the refrigerator for several weeks.

INFUSED GINGER, LAVENDER, OR CINNAMON-CARDAMOM SIMPLE SYRUP

YIELD: about 15 to 16 ounces (465 to 480 ml)	**TARGET DOSE:** 16 mg CBD | 4 mg THC per ounce (30 ml) (using a flower infusion)

EQUIPMENT
Digital scale
Peeler
Measuring cups
Measuring spoons
Small saucepan
Thermometer
One 16-ounce (480-ml)
    sterilized Mason jar
Cheesecloth
Fine-mesh strainer

INGREDIENTS
**3 grams decarboxylated
    flower of your choice**
2 cups (480 ml) water
1 cup (340 g) honey
**1½ heaping tablespoons
    sliced peeled fresh ginger
    (*for other herbs and
    spices, see note below)**
**1 tablespoon (15 ml) food-
    grade vegetable glycerin**

Weigh 3 grams of decarboxylated flower. Set aside.

Combine the water, honey, and ginger in a small saucepan. Bring to a soft boil, stirring until the honey dissolves into the water. Reduce the heat to around 160°F to 180°F (71°C to 82°C) and add the decarboxylated cannabis.

Simmer over low heat for 50 minutes, stirring occasionally. Reduce the heat and add the vegetable glycerin—this will give the CBD (and THC) something to bind to. Continue to heat and stir for 10 minutes. Remove from the heat.

Pour the infused simple syrup into a 16-ounce (480-ml) Mason jar through cheesecloth placed in a fine-mesh strainer to remove the solids. Let cool and shake before serving.

Store in the refrigerator for several weeks.

IMPORTANT: *Different honeys will produce different aroms and flavors. For this recipe, I used a mild honey with citrus and floral notes.*

NOTE

To make lavender simple syrup, simply substitute the ginger for 3 table-spoons (8 g) organic food-grade dried lavender flowers, then proceed with the recipe as noted. To make cinnamon-cardamom simple syrup, simply substitute the ginger for 1 tablespoon (2 g) whole semi-cracked cardamom pods and 4 cinnamon sticks, then proceed with the recipe as noted.

FULL-SPECTRUM INFUSED HONEY

If you're a fan of hot drinks, smoothies, or shakes, having infused honey on hand is a reliable way to incorporate CBD and THC into a variety of beverages. To create your own, all you need are a few essential ingredients: unflavored full-spectrum hemp CBD or cannabis oil, honey, and optional liquid sunflower lecithin to help prevent the oil from separating out. Simply blend the ingredients together, and voilà! You've made cannabis-infused honey.

YIELD: 1 cup (320 g)	**TARGET DOSE:** about 5 mg CBD | < 1 mg THC per teaspoon or your preferred dose (using commercially made CBD/THC oil or tincture of your choice)

EQUIPMENT
Measuring spoons
Measuring cups
Blender
One 8-ounce (240-ml)
 sterilized Mason jar

INGREDIENTS
1 tablespoon (15 ml)
 unflavored full-spectrum
 hemp or cannabis oil of
 your choice (240 mg
 CBD \| 30 mg THC or
 your preferred dose)
1 cup (320 g) honey
1 teaspoon liquid sunflower
 lecithin (optional)

Add the full-spectrum cannabis oil, honey, and liquid sunflower lecithin (if using) to a blender. Blend on high speed for a couple of minutes, then empty the infused honey into an 8-ounce (240-ml) Mason jar. Seal tightly, then let your infused honey settle for 24 hours, giving it a good stir before serving. If separation occurs over time, re-emulsify by blending the honey again or vigorously mixing with a spoon.

NOTE

If you're using THC-rich oil with this recipe, be sure to calculate the estimated dose per serving and use a teaspoon to precisely dose. You can also infuse honey using decarboxylated flower and the stovetop method, but this technique takes much longer and is a stickier process for infusion.

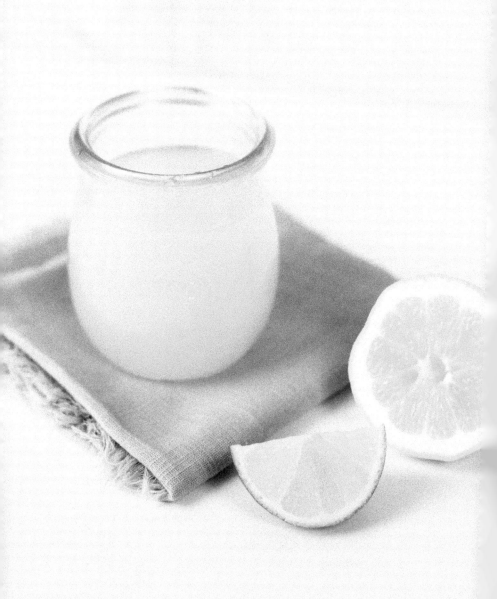

INFUSED SOUR MIX

To add sour flavors to your drinks, CBD sour mix is a must-have bar pantry item. Providing a perfect balance for overly sweet ingredients, sour mix can add dimension, livening up the flavors of your drinks so they play nicely on your palate. Combining fresh squeezed lemon and lime juice with a hint of Infused Rich Simple Syrup (page 89), this recipe works best when infusing margaritas, pisco sours, and more.

YIELD: about 20 ounces (591 ml)	**TARGET DOSE:** 3 mg CBD | 1 mg THC per ounce (30 ml) (using Infused Rich Simple Syrup, page 89)

EQUIPMENT
Citrus juicer
Fine-mesh strainer
One 32-ounce (960-ml)
    sterilized Mason jar

INGREDIENTS
1 cup (240 ml) fresh
    squeezed lemon juice
    (about 4 large lemons)
1 cup (240 ml) fresh
    squeezed lime juice
    (8 or 9 limes)
½ cup (120 ml) Infused Rich
    Simple Syrup (page 89;
    use only a ¼ cup [60 ml]
    if you prefer more sour
    than sweet flavors)

Pour the lemon and lime juices through a fine-mesh strainer into a 32-ounce (960-ml) Mason jar to remove seeds, pulp, and pith. Add the infused rich simple syrup. Seal the Mason jar tightly and shake the mixture vigorously. Store in the refrigerator and use within 1 to 2 weeks for the freshest flavor.

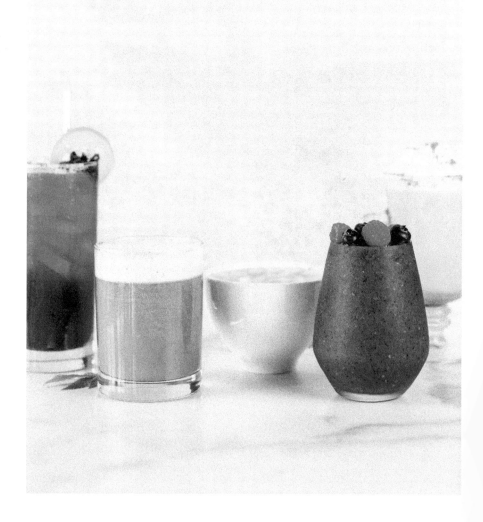

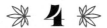

COFFEE, TEA, JUICES, SHAKES, AND SMOOTHIES

Whether you're looking for a healing protein shake to enjoy after a big work-out, an infused tea to calm the mind, or a delicious coffee or fruit smoothie to boost your energy, this chapter has it all.

When preparing hot drinks, remember to be sensitive to high heat to best preserve phytocannabinoids and terpene profiles (flip to page 64 for a temperature guide). Never boil your cannabis-infused ingredients and always keep a close eye on cooking temperatures while crafting warm infused beverages at home.

As a reminder, I used Cannatonic flower to craft the DIY infusions, which measured at a total of 12 percent CBD and 3 percent THC before decarboxylation, to determine the target dose. These numbers will differ depending on the strain and source of the product you use, so be sure to calculate your own CBD/THC milligrams per serving before making your infusion (refer to page 33). While the recipes in this section call for DIY infusions to enhance the drinks, you can easily add CBD or THC into each recipe using a commercially made unflavored tincture at your preferred dose.

Are you ready to craft cannabis-infused drinks? Don't worry. You've got this! I hope you love this selection of easy-to-make beverages.

COFFEE AND TEA

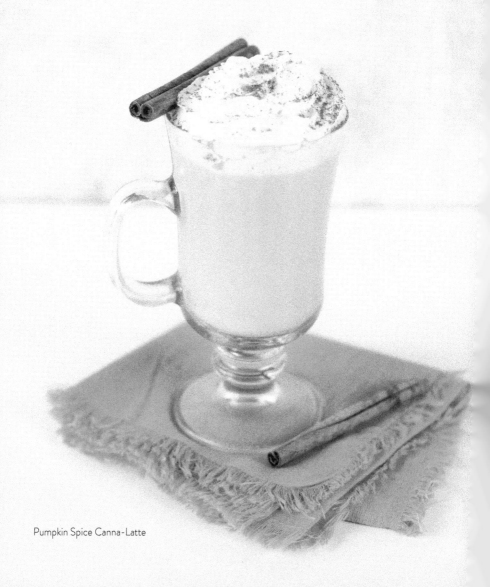

Pumpkin Spice Canna-Latte

PUMPKIN SPICE CANNA-LATTE

As fall approaches, there's something so satisfying about enjoying a pumpkin spice latte. Harmoniously combining the flavors of cinnamon, nutmeg, allspice, and ginger with smooth pumpkin purée, this autumn classic just got even better with the addition of CBD and THC! I crave this recipe all year long, especially on chillier days when I'm in need of a hot drink. If you're a pumpkin spice lover, this recipe is sure to hit the spot!

YIELD: 1 serving	**TARGET DOSE:** 10 to 15 mg CBD | 1 to 2 mg THC per drink (using Full-Spectrum Infused Honey, page 91) or your preferred dose (using commercially made CBD or THC tincture of your choice, see note below)

EQUIPMENT
Measuring cups
Measuring spoons
Small saucepan
Whisk
Coffee mug
Spoon

INGREDIENTS
2 ounces (60 ml) hot espresso or bold coffee (Add more if you prefer a stronger coffee.)
¾ cup (177 ml) milk of your choice (I prefer 2% dairy milk with this recipe.)
4 tablespoons (61 g) canned pumpkin purée
¼ teaspoon vanilla extract
½ teaspoon pumpkin pie spice blend
2 to 3 teaspoons (14 to 21 g) Full-Spectrum Infused Honey (page 91) (Add more if you prefer a sweeter taste.)

Whipped cream and a sprinkle of ground cinnamon and ground nutmeg (optional)

While the espresso is brewing, combine the milk with the pumpkin purée, vanilla, pumpkin spice blend, and infused honey to taste in a small saucepan. Warm over medium heat. Slowly whisk until the mixture is blended well. Remove from the heat. Pour the brewed espresso into a coffee cup, then slowly pour in the infused pumpkin spice milk to combine. Stir together with a spoon. Top with whipped cream and a sprinkle of cinnamon and nutmeg (if using) for enhanced aromatics and flavor.

NOTE: *If you don't have the supplies to infuse CBD or THC into the honey, simply substitute non-infused honey and add your favorite unflavored tincture (at your preferred dose) to the mug before topping with the warmed pumpkin milk. Use a spoon to mix the ingredients together, then proceed with the recipe.*

COFFEE AND TEA

THE BENEFITS OF CANNABIS +
COFFEE

featuring Christopher Schroeder & Clayton Coker, founders of Sōmatik

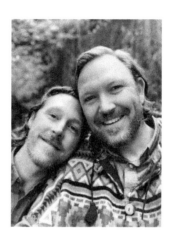

Christopher Schroeder and Clayton Coker are experts when it comes to cannabis and coffee. Established in 2016, their company, Sōmatik, is on a mission to make plant-based wellness easy to love and accessible to all. Their magic edibles and drinkables are handcrafted with adaptogens to give the body what it needs to find mind-body balance. Based in San Francisco, California, Sōmatik combines science and craft to develop plant-based medicines from vegan, organic ingredients. From infused coffee to chocolate-covered "Sparks," Christopher and Clayton are passionate about combining superfoods and herbal medicines to soothe pain and anxiety. Follow Christopher and Clayton @besomatik and @somatikwellness or visit www.somatik.us.

CHRISTOPHER SCHROEDER & CLAYTON COKER: "Have you ever tried coffee and cannabis? The effects of this pair are really quite delightful! We love the way both are rooted in long-standing social rituals, and together, they create a truly unique experience that's one part science, one part synergy.

The flavor notes of coffee and cannabis are terpene-heavy and very complementary. Both plants often have citrus notes with a fruity, robust smell. But this combination creates more than just a great tasting drink. From our research, caffeine and CBD create harmony in the brain's neuroreceptors in a way that exceeds the sum of the parts, enhancing your brain's ability to fully utilize your serotonin.

This combination can provide an elevated mood boost that's focused and euphoric. You'll likely be more aware of your breath, being able to balance both your mind and body. Despite how counterintuitive this combination might sound, we believe it's effective at reducing stress and anxiety while grounding you more deeply, the perfect combination for yoga and other self-care routines.

There's really no bad way to enjoy coffee. Whether sipping an infused coffee-based mocktail for a midday pick-me-up or kick-starting your morning with a warm coffee drink, here are a few of our go-to recipes that you can easily assemble at home."

ICED CREAMY MYLK LATTE

YIELD: **1** serving

TARGET DOSE: 2.5 mg CBD | 2.5 mg THC per iced latte (using Sōmatik Cold Brew) or 7.5 mg CBD | 2 mg THC per iced latte (using Infused Rich Simple Syrup, page 89)

EQUIPMENT
Shaker tin
Old-fashioned glass

INGREDIENTS
2 ounces (60 ml) Sōmatik CBD-infused cold brew or cold brew of your choice

4 ounces (120 ml) nut mylk (Ripple or milk substitute of your choice)

1 ounce (30 ml) cassava syrup or ½ ounce (15 ml) Infused Rich Simple Syrup (page 89)

Ice

Freshly grated nutmeg and a fresh mint leaf, for garnish

Add the cold brew, nut mylk, and syrup to a shaker tin and shake with ice. Pour into an old-fashioned cocktail glass, then top with a dusting of freshly grated nutmeg and a mint leaf. We love this drink because the fat from the nut mylk gives you a delectable latte flavor that's completely plant-based!

5-LEAF FIZZ

YIELD: **1** serving

TARGET DOSE: 5 mg CBD | 5 mg THC per iced latte (using Sōmatik Cold Brew) or 4 mg CBD | 1 mg THC per iced latte (using Infused Rich Simple Syrup, page 89)

EQUIPMENT
Shaker tin
Highball glass

INGREDIENTS
4 ounces (120 ml) Sōmatik CBD-infused cold brew or cold brew of your choice
1½ ounces (45 ml) tart cherry juice
Juice of ½ lemon
½ ounce (15 ml) cassava syrup, or ¼ ounce Infused Rich Simple Syrup (page 89)
Ice
Soda water
Lemon wheel and rosemary sprig, for garnish

In a shaker tin, shake the cold brew, cherry juice, lemon juice, and syrup. Pour into a highball glass filled with fresh cubed ice and top with soda water. Add a lemon wheel and sprig of rosemary, then enjoy.

COFFEE AND TEA

DAILY BONUS (ADD A SHOT!)

Much like a classic "add shot" with new heights, this daily bonus gives your morning brew an extra kick of caffeine—and an added stress buffer on your way to work! Simply prepare 8 ounces (240 ml) of hot coffee to your liking. Pour in 1 to 2 ounces (30 to 60 ml) of cannabis-infused cold brew, then enjoy!

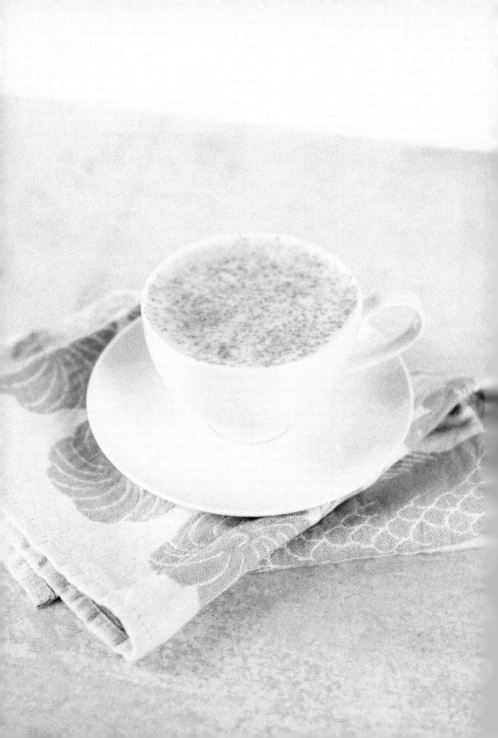

TURMERIC LATTE

As an alternative to traditional coffee drinks, an uplifting turmeric latte is a great way to add extra antioxidants into your diet. Packed with powerful anti-inflammatory properties, a portion of turmeric's healing powers come from curcumin, which is the herb's main active ingredient derived from curcuminoids. Curcumin neutralize free radicals and it's also linked to enhanced brain function. With the addition of Full-Spectrum Infused Honey (page 91), this power team is loaded with therapeutic benefits. If you've never tasted a turmeric latte, this healthy drink might become your new morning go-to!

YIELD: 1 serving	**TARGET DOSE:** 10 mg CBD | 1.25 mg THC (using Full-Spectrum Infused Honey, page 91) or your preferred dose (using commercially made CBD or THC tincture of your choice, see note below)

EQUIPMENT
Small saucepan
Whisk
Single-serve blender
Latte cup

INGREDIENTS
1 cup (240 ml) milk of your choice (I prefer coconut milk with this recipe.)

½ teaspoon ground turmeric

¼ teaspoon ground cinnamon

⅛ teaspoon ground ginger

¼ teaspoon vanilla extract

2 teaspoons (14 g) Full-Spectrum Infused Honey (page 91. Add more if you prefer a sweeter taste.)

Turmeric powder, for garnish

In a small saucepan, warm the milk over medium heat, stirring, for 2 to 3 minutes, or until hot but not boiling. Reduce the heat and add the spices, vanilla, and infused honey. Use a whisk to blend the ingredients well, creating a slight froth, then remove from the heat. Transfer the infused turmeric milk into a single-serve blender and blend on high speed for 10 seconds, creating extra froth for the latte. Pour the turmeric latte into a latte cup, add a sprinkle of turmeric powder on top, and enjoy.

NOTE: *If you don't have the supplies to infuse CBD or THC into the honey, simply substitute regular honey and add your favorite unflavored tincture (at your preferred dose) into the blender before blending the ingredients together, then proceed with the recipe.*

COFFEE AND TEA

CBD BUTTER COFFEE

Butter coffee tastes delicious and it's also keto-friendly, supporting a high-fat, low-carb diet. Because butter is a rich source of fat, it's been known to slow digestion, evoking the feeling of being full. I personally love butter coffee for its richness on the palate. It's so smooth and silky, plus you don't need to add a bunch of cream or sugar to alter the flavor.

YIELD: **1** serving	**TARGET DOSE:** your preferred dose (using commercially made full-spectrum CBD MCT oil of your choice or your DIY Infused MCT tincture, see recipe below)

EQUIPMENT
Coffee maker
Small saucepan
Single-serve blender
Measuring spoons
Coffee mug

INGREDIENTS
1 cup (240 ml) hot brewed coffee, made your preferred way

1½ tablespoons (21 g) grass-fed European-style butter

1 teaspoon CBD MCT oil tincture (or your preferred dose; your favorite brand or opposite)

½ teaspoon organic cacao powder

¾ ounce (22 ml) coconut milk, for extra froth (optional)

Once the coffee is brewed, add the hot coffee to a single-serve blender, then add the butter, CBD MCT oil, cacao powder, and coconut milk (if using). Blend on high speed for 10 seconds, making sure the mixture is extra creamy. Pour into a large coffee mug and enjoy.

HOW TO MAKE AN INFUSED MCT OIL TINCTURE AT HOME

Weigh 7 grams of decarboxylated flower of your choice. In a 16-ounce (480-ml) Mason jar, combine the flower with ¾ cup (180 ml) MCT oil. Seal the top tightly. Fill the bottom of a small saucepan with water. Set the Mason jar inside and begin to heat over medium-low heat; the water should not go to the top of the Mason jar. Continue to heat until you reach a gentle boil (around 200°F [93°C]), then cook for 2 hours, making sure the water does not exceed 211°F (99°C). Check frequently and refill the saucepan with water as needed due to evaporation. When finished, remove the Mason jar safely with an oven mitt and let the jar cool. Place a cheesecloth in a fine-mesh strainer. Pour the infused MCT oil over the cheesecloth into a clean 8-ounce (240-ml) Mason jar. Double filter if needed for clarity, then funnel into a glass bottle with a dropper cap. Store at room temperature in a dark cabinet. It will stay fresh for several months if stored properly.

SUMMER BERRY PALMER

Part iced tea, part lemonade, the Arnold Palmer is a celebrated summer
favorite that's undeniably refreshing. Originating in the late 1960s, this
thirst-quenching concoction was named after world-famous golfer, Arnold
Palmer, after he ordered the combination after a long day on the golf
course. I love making Arnold Palmers, especially with a twist! I call this
recipe the Summer Berry Palmer. Blending freshly prepared raspberry
iced tea, fresh cannabis-infused lemonade, and muddled raspberries and
blackberries, this is the perfect alcohol-free drink to quench your thirst.

YIELD: 1 serving	TARGET DOSE: 7 mg CBD | 2 mg THC per drink (using Cannabis-Infused Lemonade, page 108) or your preferred dose (using commercially made CBD or THC tincture of your choice, see note below)

EQUIPMENT
Small saucepan
One 8-ounce (240-ml)
    sterilized Mason jar
Shaker tin
Muddler
Fine-mesh strainer
Highball glass
Bar spoon

INGREDIENTS
1 cup (240 ml) water
2 raspberry tea bags
Ice
4 or 5 fresh raspberries
4 or 5 fresh blackberries
5 ounces (150 ml) Cannabis-
    infused Lemonade
    (recipe page 108)
Fresh berries, a lemon wheel,
    and a thyme sprig, for
    garnish

Begin by brewing the raspberry tea. Using a small
saucepan, bring the water to a boil, then remove
from the heat. Add the teabags and steep for
4 minutes. Remove the teabags, then pour the
raspberry tea into an 8-ounce (240-ml) Mason jar
and set in the refrigerator to cool.

Once chilled, fill a highball glass with ice, then add
the raspberries and blackberries to the shaker tin.
Muddle the fruit together until the juices release,
then add 5 ounces (150 ml) of the chilled raspberry
tea. Cover and dry shake (no ice) vigorously for 10
seconds, then strain the liquid through a fine-mesh
strainer into the highball glass. Add the cannabis-
infused lemonade, then stir together using a bar
spoon. Add fresh berries, lemon wheel, and thyme
sprig to garnish.

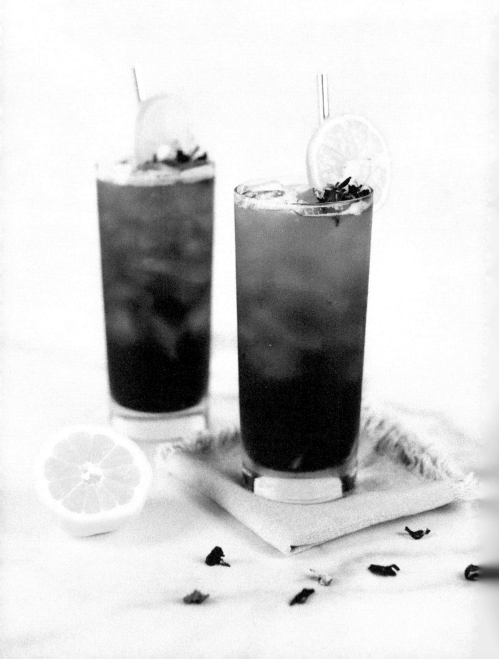

HOT & COLD GINGER, LEMON, HIBISCUS-INFUSED TEA

Whether you're a hot tea lover or crave a refreshing glass of iced tea, this recipe is packed with healing herbs to help keep your body balanced. If you're feeling a bit under the weather, I recommend enjoying this recipe hot as the ginger, lemon, and hibiscus provide unique therapeutic benefits that will help you feel better in no time.

YIELD: 1 serving	**TARGET DOSE:** 8 mg CBD | 2 mg THC per drink (using Infused Ginger Simple Syrup, page 90) or your preferred dose (using commercially made CBD or THC tincture of your choice, see note below)

EQUIPMENT
Small saucepan
Teacup or mug
Fine-mesh strainer
Teaspoon

INGREDIENTS
1 cup (240 ml) water
1 teaspoon thinly sliced peeled fresh ginger
1 or 2 hibiscus tea bags
½ ounce (15 ml) Infused Ginger Simple Syrup (page 90), ¼ ounce if you prefer less sweet
1 ounce (30 ml) fresh squeezed lemon juice
Lemon wedges and hibiscus leaves, for garnish

In a small saucepan, bring the water and ginger to a boil. Remove from the heat, then add the tea bags. Let steep for 10 minutes, or until the water has turned a dark pink color.

Remove the tea bags and reheat if the liquid has cooled. While the tea is reheating, add the infused simple syrup and lemon juice to the bottom of a teacup. Remove the tea from heat and use a fine-mesh strainer to separate the liquid from the solids over the mug. Use a teaspoon to stir the mixture together, then add a lemon wedge and hibiscus leaves to garnish.

Flip to page 108 for the cold Ginger, Lemon, Hibiscus-Infused Tea recipe.

COFFEE AND TEA

NOTE

If you don't have the supplies to infuse the simple syrup with CBD or THC, substitute regular simple syrup, then add your favorite unflavored tincture (at your preferred dose) into the mug (hot) or shaker tin (cold), then follow the directions as written.

HOW TO MAKE COLD GINGER, LEMON, HIBISCUS-INFUSED TEA

To make a chilled iced tea, follow the directions on page 107, but after you remove the hibiscus tea bags, let the ginger hibiscus tea cool to room temperature. Once cool, add the ginger hibiscus tea, infused simple syrup, and fresh squeezed lemon juice to a shaker tin with ice. Shake vigorously for 15 seconds or until very cold. Strain over a glass of your choice filled with fresh ice, then garnish with a lemon wedge and hibiscus leaves.

HOW TO MAKE CANNABIS-INFUSED LEMONADE

YIELD: 11 ounces (330 ml)

Using a citrus juicer, juice 1 cup (240 ml) of fresh squeezed lemon juice. Remove the seeds and keep the pulp. Pour the lemon juice into a mixing bowl, then add 1 ounce (30 ml) of Infused Rich Simple Syrup (page 89) and 2 ounces (60 ml) non-infused rich simple syrup. Use a whisk to blend the ingredients together, then taste the lemonade. If you prefer a sweeter taste, add more non-infused rich simple syrup (or Infused Rich Simple Syrup, page 89, for a stronger dose), then whisk again. You can either enjoy this infused lemonade by itself over ice or transfer it to a Mason jar and chill in the refrigerator until further use. If you don't have the supplies to infuse the rich simple syrup, simply substitute regular rich simple syrup, then add your favorite unflavored tincture (at your preferred dose) into the mixing bowl before whisking. Follow the directions as written and shake vigorously before serving.

MASALA CHAI CANNABIS TEA

Spicy with a hint of sweet, masala chai tea is a brilliant blend of black tea, savory spices, and milk. This uplifting hot drink is a fantastic alternative to coffee, containing caffeine, which is derived from black tea leaves. There are many ways to prepare this popular beverage; however, to make it a masala chai, you must incorporate an array of spices cooked over heat for the best concentration of flavors. This recipe is also incredibly easy to infuse with the addition of Full-Spectrum Infused Honey (page 91). Get ready to cozy up with this warm and comforting cannabis tea drink.

YIELD: 1 serving	**TARGET DOSE:** 7.5 to 10 mg CBD | < 1 to 1.25 mg THC per drink (using Full-Spectrum Infused Honey, page 91) or your preferred dose (using commercially made CBD or THC tincture of your choice, see note below)

EQUIPMENT
Small saucepan
Fine-mesh strainer
Large coffee mug

INGREDIENTS
¾ cup (180 ml) water
1 teaspoon thinly sliced peeled fresh ginger
½ teaspoon black peppercorns, crushed
2 cinnamon sticks
2 or 3 whole cloves, crushed
5 cracked cardamom pods
¾ cup (180 ml) milk of your choice (I prefer coconut milk.)
2 black tea bags

1½ to 2 teaspoons Full-Spectrum Infused Honey (page 91)
Cinnamon stick, for garnish

Combine the water, ginger, peppercorns, cinnamon sticks, cloves, and cardamom pods in a small saucepan. Warm over medium heat until the water begins to boil, stirring occasionally. Reduce the heat and simmer for 10 minutes. Remove from the heat.

Add the milk of your choice, stir together with the other ingredients, then add the black tea bags. Steep for 5 minutes, agitating the tea bags from time to time, then remove and discard the bags. Begin to heat the chai tea once again over low heat until warm. Using a fine-mesh strainer, separate the solids from the liquid over a large coffee mug, then stir in the infused honey to taste until it dissolves. Add a cinnamon stick to garnish, then serve immediately.

COFFEE AND TEA

NOTE *If you don't have the supplies to make infused honey, simply substitute regular honey and add your favorite unflavored tincture (at your preferred dose) into the coffee mug when the honey is added, then proceed with the recipe.*

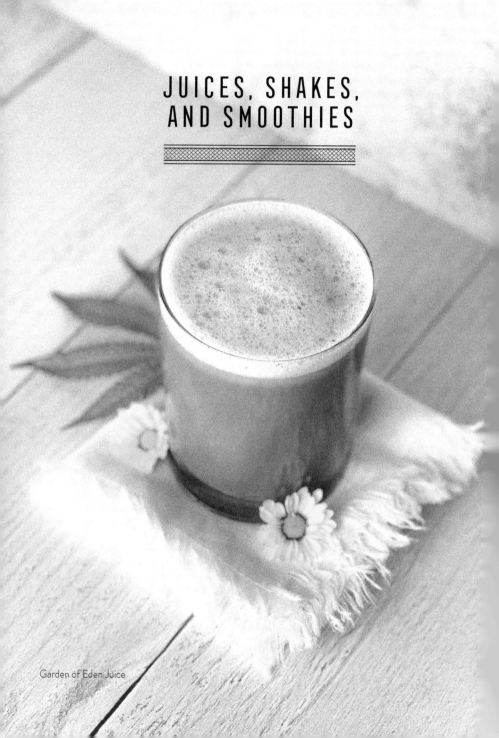

JUICES, SHAKES, AND SMOOTHIES

Garden of Eden Juice

GARDEN OF EDEN JUICE

If you're craving a delicious green juice, but don't have a juicer at home, this recipe is for you! Garden of Eden can be made using only a blender and a fine-mesh strainer. Incorporating a mixture of leafy greens, vegetables, herbs, and fruits, this supercharged juice provides a boost of nutrients as well as THCA and CBDA, the primary nonintoxicating phytocannabinoids that you'll find in fresh cannabis leaves. Blend this up in the morning to jumpstart your system.

YIELD: 1 serving	**TARGET DOSE**: Nonintoxicating CBDA and THCA

EQUIPMENT
Blender
Fine-mesh strainer
One 8-ounce (240-ml)
   drinking glass

INGREDIENTS
1 cup (240 ml) water

1 apple, sliced

2 slices unpeeled lemon

5 whole kale leaves

1 (1-inch or 2.5-cm) piece
   fresh ginger, peeled

3 celery stalks, cut in half

3 large fresh cannabis leaves
   (or spinach or dandelion
   leaves)

1 cup ice

Add the water to the blender. Layer in your ingredients on top of the water. The last thing you'll add is ice. Once the blender is full, purée on high speed for 2 minutes.

Using a fine-mesh strainer, separate the juice from the pulp over an 8-ounce (240-ml) drinking glass. The pulp is thick, and you might need to empty the pulp from the strainer a few times to best capture the juice. Continue this process until the glass is filled with your newly created green juice. Enjoy!

NOTE

I like my green juices extra "green" tasting. If you'd like to add more sweetness, add 1 teaspoon of infused honey or a few slices of pineapple to this recipe before blending. The best way to source fresh cannabis leaves is to grow your own plants; however, if you cannot access fresh cannabis leaves, you can simply use other leafy greens to enhance this recipe.

THE BENEFITS OF JUICING CANNABIS

featuring Erin Willis, holistic nutritionist, cannabis educator
& creator of Mother Indica

Erin Willis is a holistic nutritionist, cannabis educator, and writer. She believes that all energies and ecological systems are connected and that utilizing and flowing with the natural world is our answer to a thriving, balanced society. Erin has made it her life's mission to help shift the disease-causing status quo of the Western world by debunking cannabis misconceptions, encouraging a botanical-based lifestyle, and helping pave the way for a modern, integrative health paradigm. For a deep dive into holistic nutrition and plant medicine, follow Erin @mother_indica or be sure to visit www.motherindica.com.

ERIN WILLIS: "With achieving health and vitality, many modalities can feel overwhelming. We've all been there. Sleeping past our alarm clock, waking up with a groggy body and mind, brain fog clouding our thoughts, and our joints achy and inflamed. Not the most inspiring way to start the day. For me, this is where the dynamic combination of cannabis and juicing comes in.

Your body can heal itself with a little help from Mother Nature. Many plants, including cannabis, can give you the tools your body needs to slide back into a balanced, functioning state. These tools come in the form of micro- and macronutrients and microorganisms. Including live water, raw enzymes, electrolytes, trace minerals, vitamins, healthy fatty acids, and essential amino acids. All essential components that work in synergy to revitalize your natural systems. Adding phytocannabinoids, such as THCA, THC, and CBD, to your juices can be an added benefit to nourish your endocannabinoid system—an endogenous network intertwined within your digestive and immune systems.

A simple way to consume this long list of elements? With a daily cannabis-infused green juice. Frequently juicing fresh, organic greens and low-glycemic fruits means your body gets to gently absorb a plethora of raw, nutrient-dense vegetables, fruits, leafy greens, and herbs. Flooding your beautiful body with alkalizing, detoxifying, and energizing plant medicines."

GREEN GOODNESS CANNABIS JUICE

YIELD: 1 serving

TARGET DOSE: 10 to 15 mg CBD | 1.25 to 2 mg THC per drink (using Full-Spectrum Infused Honey, page 91)

EQUIPMENT
Juicer

INGREDIENTS
3 handfuls fresh cannabis leaves or kale, spinach, or dandelion leaves

1 head romaine lettuce

2 cucumbers

5 celery stalks, leaves removed

1 cup (70 g) tightly packed fresh parsley

1 lemon, peeled and cut in half

1 (½-inch or 1-cm) piece fresh ginger, peeled and sliced in half

½ to 1 tablespoon (10 to 21 g) Full-Spectrum Infused Honey (page 91)

Feed all the ingredients into a juicer, altering the romaine and celery with the leafy greens and parsley. Serve immediately with a drizzle of raw cannabis-infused honey. Feel the effects of gratitude, calm, and clarity within 30 to 120 minutes.

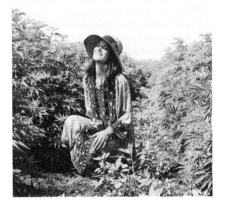

SUPERFOOD SMOOTHIE

Packed with nutrient-dense ingredients, this smoothie is one of my go-to recipes to make in the morning because it replenishes the body and provides a boost of antioxidants, fiber, and vitamins. This smoothie is seriously good for you and it's filling, acting as a meal on its own. With a line-up of unique ingredients, it's incredibly complex and scrumptious. For best results, use frozen fruit (including frozen spinach) to guarantee a thick and creamy texture.

YIELD: 1 serving	TARGET DOSE: 5 mg CBD | < 1 mg THC per smoothie (using Full-Spectrum Infused Honey, page 91) or your preferred dose (using commercially made CBD or THC tincture of your choice, see note below)

EQUIPMENT
Blender
Glass of your choice

INGREDIENTS
½ cup (127 g) frozen strawberries
¼ cup (38 g) frozen blueberries
1 small frozen banana
½ cup (30 g) frozen spinach
½ cup (120 ml) fresh squeezed orange juice
¼ cup (60 ml) pomegranate juice
1 teaspoon Full-Spectrum Infused Honey (page 91)

1½ teaspoons acai berry powder
1 teaspoon ground flaxseed
1 teaspoon organic cacao nibs
¼ teaspoon ground ginger
¼ teaspoon ground cinnamon
⅛ teaspoon black pepper

Add all the ingredients to a blender. Blend until smooth and creamy, then serve in a glass of your choice.

NOTE

If you don't have time to make infused honey, you can still incorporate CBD and THC into this recipe by adding your favorite unflavored tincture (at your preferred dose) into the blender. Simply blend with the other ingredients called for and enjoy.

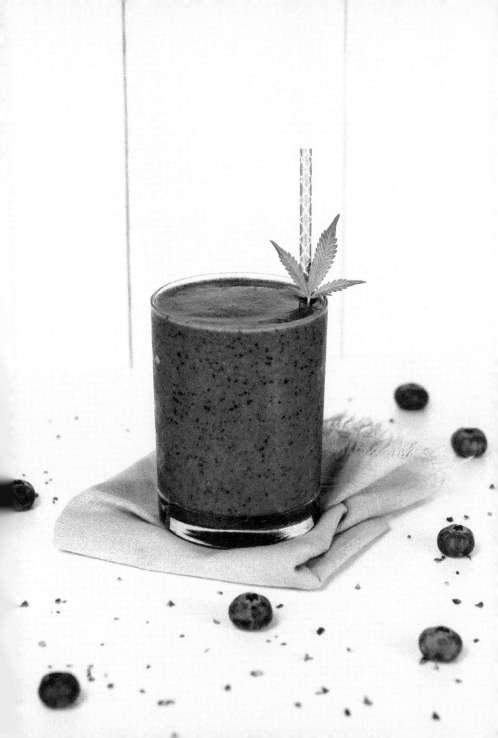

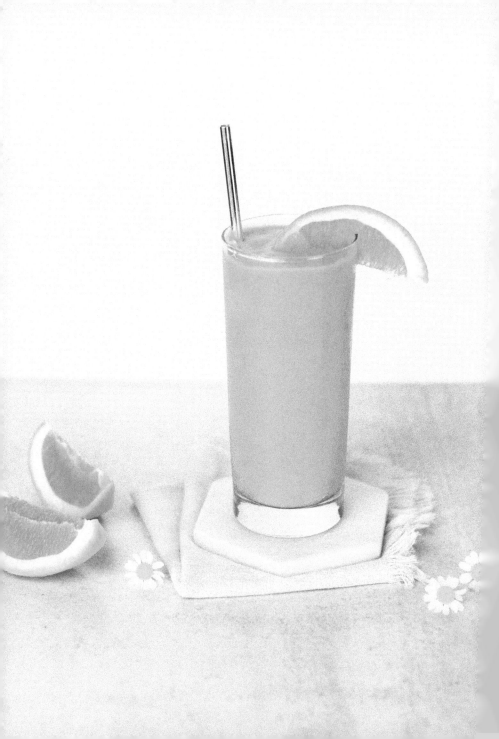

VITAMIN CBD IMMUNITY SMOOTHIE

As flu season approaches, this smoothie is just what the doctor ordered. Naturally packed with vitamin C and Full-Spectrum Infused Honey (page 91), this delicious, energizing drink will jumpstart your immune system, helping fight off a number of ailments. One of the most power-packed ingredients included is camu camu. If you're new to this superfood, it's known to contain almost ten times more vitamin C than a single orange. That's potent! For best results, use frozen fruits in this recipe. Your end results will be sorbet-like, so don't be afraid to eat this with a spoon.

YIELD: 1 serving	**TARGET DOSE:** 5 mg CBD | < 1 mg THC per smoothie (using Full-Spectrum Infused Honey, page 91) or your preferred dose (using commercially made CBD or THC tincture of your choice, see note below)

EQUIPMENT
Blender
Glass of your choice

INGREDIENTS
½ cup (85 g) frozen pineapple
½ cup (90 g) frozen mango
1 small frozen banana
½ cup (120 ml) fresh–pressed carrot juice
¼ cup (60 ml) fresh squeezed orange juice

1 teaspoon Full-Spectrum Infused Honey (page 91)
1 teaspoon fresh squeezed lemon juice
1 teaspoon camu camu powder
¼ teaspoon ground ginger
Fresh orange slice, for garnish

Add all the ingredients to a blender. Blend until smooth and creamy. Serve in a glass of your choice, and garnish with a slice of orange.

NOTE

If you don't have time to make infused honey, you can still incorporate CBD and THC into this recipe by adding your favorite unflavored tincture (at your preferred dose) into the blender. Simply blend with the other ingredients called for and enjoy.

CHOCOLATE BANANA
PROTEIN SHAKE

If you're a fitness enthusiast, this infused Chocolate Banana Protein Shake is the perfect beverage to replenish your body. Allowing worn-out muscles to recover, while providing healthy nutrients and anti-inflammatory properties, add this delicious shake to your post-workout routine to keep your mind and body feeling balanced. Plus, who doesn't love chocolate?!

YIELD: 1 serving	**TARGET DOSE:** your preferred dose (using commercially made CBD or THC tincture of your choice)

EQUIPMENT
Blender
Glass of your choice

INGREDIENTS
1 frozen banana

1½ tablespoons (9 g) raw cacao powder

1 scoop low-sugar vanilla protein powder

1 tablespoon (7 g) hemp hearts, plus more for serving

1 heaping teaspoon raw cacao nibs

¼ teaspoon ground cinnamon

6 ounces (180 ml) milk of your choice (I prefer nondairy milk with this recipe.)

CBD or THC tincture of your choice (at your preferred dose)

Add all the ingredients to a blender. Blend until thick and creamy, then pour into a drinking glass of your choice to serve. Sprinkle with hemp hearts to add extra crunch.

PB & J PROTEIN SHAKE

Who doesn't love the classic flavor combination of peanut butter and jelly! This spin on the old childhood classic is packed with protein and nutrients, making it a fantastic go-to in the morning or after your workout routine. Offering a perfect blend of salty and sweet flavors, plus a healing dose of CBD and/or THC, this shake is a delicious way to start the day, plus will help battle inflammation.

YIELD: 1 serving	**TARGET DOSE:** your preferred dose (using commercially made CBD or THC tincture of your choice)

EQUIPMENT
Blender
Glass of your choice

INGREDIENTS
1 frozen banana

1 cup (145 g) mixed frozen berries

1 tablespoon (16 g) organic unsalted peanut butter

1 tablespoon (20 g) raspberry jelly or jelly of your choice

1 scoop low-sugar vanilla protein powder

1 tablespoon (6 g) oats

1 cup (240 ml) milk of your choice

CBD or THC tincture of your choice (at your preferred dose)

Crushed peanuts and fresh berries of your choice, for garnish (optional)

Combine the frozen banana, frozen berries, peanut butter, raspberry jelly, protein powder, oats, milk, and unflavored tincture of your choice in a blender. Blend until smooth. Pour into a drinking glass of your choice. Top with crushed peanuts and fresh berries (if using), then serve immediately.

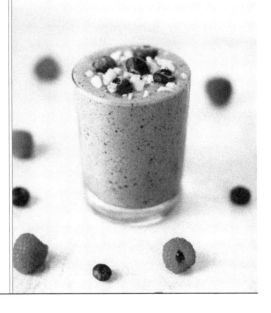

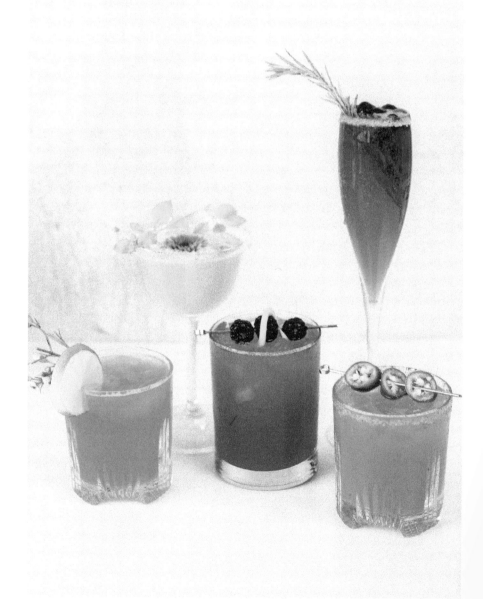

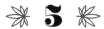
SPIRIT-FREE MIXED DRINKS AND COCKTAILS

As an aspiring cannabis mixologist, learning how to craft balanced and complex spirit-free mixed drinks and cocktails is the next task on your list. These recipes are more complicated than crafting infused tea, coffee, juices, shakes, and smoothies. Be sure to reference chapters 2 and 3 for a deeper understanding of mixology techniques and how to create infusions.

The recipes in this section include DIY infusions, which I made from Cannatonic flower measuring at a total of 12 percent CBD and 3 percent THC before decarboxylation to determine the target dose. These numbers will differ depending on the strain and source of the product you use, so be sure to calculate your own CBD/THC milligrams per serving before making your infusion (refer to page 33 for at-home dosage calculations). If you don't have time to make an infusion, don't worry! You can easily add CBD or THC to each recipe using your favorite unflavored tincture at your preferred dose. Refer to page 31 to review dosing recommendations.

If you're planning to use THC, be cautious when mixing with alcohol. Both cannabis and alcohol can be potent intoxicants if you consume too much, presenting negative side effects such as dizziness and upset stomach. Consuming both can also amplify sedating side effects, so it's best to keep CBD/THC dosages low (or a microdose). If you're taking other medications, it's best to play it safe. Do not mix with CBD, THC, or alcohol. And above all, do not operate machinery or drive after consuming CBD or THC cocktails. Cheers and consume responsibly!

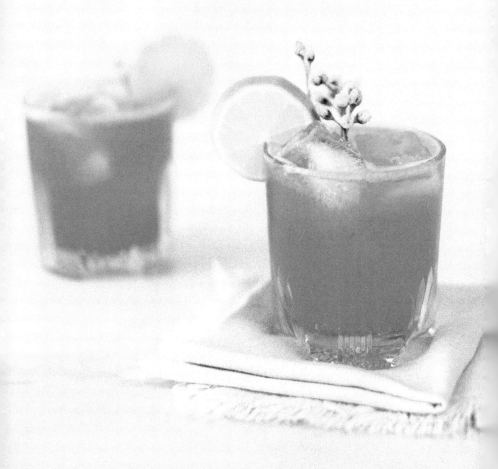

SPIRIT-FREE MIXED DRINKS

Raspberry Rickey

RASPBERRY RICKEY

Refreshingly tart with a hint of sweetness, this alcohol-free raspberry rickey is the perfect aperitif to serve before a feast with friends. Traditionally, the rickey is made with gin and lime juice with a splash of sparkling water; however, to make this a tasty spirit-free mixed cannabis drink, we will skip the gin this time and add raspberry, lime, and Infused Rich Simple Syrup (page 89) for complexity and bright flavors. I love working with raspberries, not only for the taste, but also for the beautiful pink hue they bring to a drink. This rickey is thirst-quenching and delicious!

YIELD: 1 serving	**TARGET DOSE:** 7.5 mg CBD | 2 mg THC per drink (using Infused Rich Simple Syrup, page 89) or your preferred dose (using a commercially made CBD or THC tincture of your choice, see note below)

EQUIPMENT
Shaker tin
Muddler
Fine-mesh strainer
Old-fashioned glass

INGREDIENTS
¼ cup (33 g) raspberries
1 ounce (30 ml) fresh squeezed lime juice
½ ounce (15 ml) Infused Rich Simple Syrup (page 89)
Ice
Club soda
Lime wheel and seasonal flowers, for garnish

In a shaker tin, muddle the raspberries and lime juice. Add the infused simple syrup and ice, then cover and shake for 15 seconds or until fully chilled. Using a fine-mesh strainer, separate the solids from the liquid over an old-fashioned glass filled with fresh ice. Top the drink with a splash of club soda and give it a good stir. Express the lime over the glass, then garnish with a lime wheel and seasonal flowers.

SPIRIT-FREE MIXED DRINKS

NOTE

If you don't have the supplies to infuse the Rich Simple Syrup at home, simply substitute regular rich simple syrup, then, add your favorite unflavored tincture (at your preferred dose) into the shaker tin before muddling. Follow the directions as written.

HOW TO MAKE CRUSHED ICE AT HOME

If you've been to a cocktail bar lately, you'll notice that particular drinks are made with different types of ice. This is because the type of ice that's used impacts the drink's profile. Crushed ice is essential for certain drinks, so it's important to know how to create it in the comfort of your own home. Don't worry, this process doesn't require a fancy ice machine. Here are a couple of ways you can do this using items you most likely already own.

THE BLENDER METHOD

Using a blender or food processor, add a few handfuls of ice cubes, then pulse until you have crushed ice. Be careful not to overly crush, avoiding a snow-like texture, which will melt fast! It's as simple as that. Use the ice right away or store in a zip-top bag in the freezer if you'd like to save a batch for later.

THE BAG METHOD

While not the most efficient method, you can also crush ice using a zip-top bag and a heavy item to facilitate the crushing. Simply add a few scoops of ice to a bag, seal, then use something heavy to crush the ice. I've used a rolling pin before, but any heavy item that won't get damaged will do. Just prepare yourself for a good arm workout!

NOTE: *Remember, you never want to add crushed ice to a shaker tin when mixing drinks. This will heavily dilute your beverages because of the small ice pieces that melt fast! It's best to add the crushed ice directly into a glass, then top with liquid ingredients. Also keep in mind that using quality ice matters. Most grocery stores sell bagged ice that's been filtered and clarified.*

SUMMER CRUSH

Bright pink and refreshing, the Summer Crush will quench your thirst during those hot and steamy summer evenings. Watermelon and lime perfectly combine to delight your senses as the flavors dance on your palate. Enhanced with CBD and a dash of THC, you'll be completely infatuated with this delicious summer drink.

YIELD: **1** serving	**TARGET DOSE:** 7.5 mg CBD	2 mg THC per drink (using Infused Rich Simple Syrup, page 89) or your preferred dose (using commercially made CBD or THC tincture of your choice, see note below)

EQUIPMENT
Blender or food processor
Fine-mesh strainer
One 8-ounce (240-ml)
    sterilized Mason jar
Shaker tin
Hawthorne strainer
Chilled sour glass

WATERMELON JUICE
½ small seedless watermelon

SUMMER CRUSH
1 ounce (30 ml) fresh
    squeezed lime juice
½ ounce (15 ml) Infused Rich
    Simple Syrup (page 89)
Pinch of salt
Egg white
Ice
Seasonal edible flowers, for
    garnish

To make the watermelon juice: Add the watermelon flesh to a blender or food processor. Purée for 1 minute or until the watermelon chunks turn into juice. Using a fine-mesh strainer, separate the pulp from the juice over an 8-ounce (240-ml) Mason jar. Repeat to remove all remaining pulp (save the extra juice for your next round or turn to page 150). Discard the pulp.

To make the Summer Crush: In a shaker tin, combine 3 ounces (90 ml) of watermelon juice, the lime juice, infused rich simple syrup, salt, and egg white. Cover and dry shake (no ice) for 10 seconds, then add ice and shake again for 25 seconds to create the finest froth. Strain into a chilled sour glass and garnish with seasonal flowers.

SPIRIT-FREE MIXED DRINKS

NOTE

If you don't have the supplies to infuse the rich simple syrup, simply substitute the non-infused version and add your favorite unflavored tincture (at your preferred dose) to the shaker tin before shaking. Then, proceed with the recipe.

SPARKLING ROSEMARY GREYHOUND

If you're a grapefruit lover, the Greyhound is a classic drink that typically includes only two ingredients: grapefruit juice and either gin or vodka. This time, we're skipping the booze and adding a few new ingredients to elevate this tart beverage. Instead of alcohol, the Infused Grapefruit Rosemary Shrub (page 87), fresh squeezed grapefruit juice, and a splash of club soda add a sparkling effect. This incredibly refreshing drink cleanses the palate while it quenches your thirst. Be sure to add the rosemary sugar rim for an extra pop of flavor!

YIELD: 1 serving	**TARGET DOSE**: 6 mg CBD | 1.5 mg THC per drink (using Infused Grapefruit Rosemary Shrub, page 87) or your preferred dose (using a commercially made CBD or THC tincture of your choice, see note below)

EQUIPMENT
Coffee grinder
Shallow saucer
Old-fashioned glass
Bar spoon

ROSEMARY SUGAR RIM
1 rosemary sprig
2 tablespoons (26 g) sugar
1 grapefruit slice

SPARKLING ROSEMARY GREYHOUND
Crushed ice
1½ ounces (45 ml) Infused Grapefruit Rosemary Shrub (page 87)
1 ounce (30 ml) fresh squeezed ruby red grapefruit juice, pulp removed

Club soda
Dash Angostura bitters
Rosemary sprig and slice of grapefruit, for garnish

To make the rosemary sugar rim: Remove the needles from the rosemary sprig, then put them into a clean coffee or spice grinder along with the sugar. Grind until fine. Empty the ground rosemary and sugar into a shallow saucer. Using a grapefruit slice, rim the top of an old-fashioned glass, then dip the glass into the rosemary sugar to create a sugared rim.

To make the Sparkling Rosemary Greyhound: Carefully fill an old-fashioned glass with fresh crushed ice. Add the infused shrub and grapefruit juice, then top with club soda. Add the bitters, then gently stir with a bar spoon to mix well. Garnish with a sprig of rosemary and a slice of grapefruit before serving.

CRAFTING SPIRIT-FREE MIXED DRINKS WITH CBD OIL TINCTURES

featuring Jewel Zimmer, founder & CEO of Juna

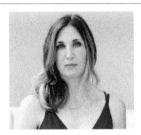

Jewel Zimmer is the founder and CEO of Juna, a premium cannabis and CBD lifestyle company that focuses on producing plant-powered tincture formulas that naturally release the body, engage the mind, enhance social situations, and tastefully integrate into every moment of daily life. With a background as a fine-dining pastry chef and certified sommelier in San Francisco, Jewel launched her first functional food, {cocoa} absolute, with Barneys New York in 2009, infusing single-origin chocolate with adaptogenic raw cacao extracts to intensify the physiological and therapeutic benefits of the fruit. The line soon gained an international following and inspired her to work with other plants and botanicals. After years of research and development, building close relationships with farmers, chemists, and medical experts, Jewel established Juna with the goal of creating targeted plant-powered formulas for mind, body, mood, and sleep. Follow Jewel and Juna @juna.world.

JEWEL ZIMMER: "At Juna, we design CBD drinks with layers of flavor, texture, and the following absolutes in mind:

Quality: Look for full-spectrum products with proven lab results and a base of MCT oil. MCT oil has a neutral flavor, it's light-bodied, meaning it will stay in your drink and NOT stick to the side of the glass, and it contributes to a clean herbal and sometimes fruity flavor. MCT is known as brain fuel. It metabolizes quickly for increased and sustained energy without the crash, jumpstarts the metabolism, decreases cravings, and supports a healthy gut microbiome. Its neutral flavor and light consistency make a perfect carrier for hemp-derived CBD as well as help support cannabidiol to work more efficiently in the body. Lastly, if taken before sleep, MCT supports hydration in the brain and works to jumpstart the brain system the next morning.

Dose: Think about how many drinks you want to serve and/or imbibe at one time, then dose accordingly. I suggest 10 milligrams of CBD per drink. If serving others, be sure to check in with your guests after one drink, then adjust the dose from there based on each guest's personal needs.

Flavor: I recommend to first taste the CBD oil, then either find a flavor combination to complement it or enhance it. For example, if it tastes like pine, try adding juniper, sage, and lavender. The next step would be to layer in a fruit. I tend to love strawberry or citrus.

PRO TIPS

A drop of salt will enhance flavor; vinegar will change the flavor, making it brighter with more depth in quality. For salt, try adding pink Himalayan.

Add texture. For me, garnish is everything: the visual; the experiential crunch of a stem; the softness of a flower petal or piece of fresh fruit. Texture is key, plus Instagram-worthy!

To make a CBD-infused drink using an MCT oil tincture, here's a recipe I've crafted for your drinking pleasure."

SPRING BOTANICAL CBD WATER

Cult Secret: For this recipe, I love using Topo Chico sparkling water because it never goes flat!

YIELD: **1** serving

TARGET DOSE: 10 mg CBD per drink using Juna "Balance Drops" or your favorite unflavored CBD tincture

---

EQUIPMENT
Old-fashioned glass

Bar spoon

SPRING BOTANICAL WITH CBD
Cubed ice

4 ounces (120 ml) sparkling mineral water

2 ounces (60 ml) Seedlip botanical garden nonalcoholic spirit

1 dropper CBD tincture (or your preferred dose)

TERPENE ADDITIONS (OPTIONAL)
1 drop limonene or lemon slice

3 drops beta-caryophyllene or crushed pink or black peppercorns

2 drops pinene or sprig rosemary and mint

GARNISHES (OPTIONAL BUT RECOMMENDED)
Crushed dried mandarin segments

Rosemary flowers

Bergamot mint or leaves

Live (hydroponic) pea tendrils

Anything alive and ready from your local farmers' market (Sage, lavender, rose, calendula, and basil are also perfect additions.)

Fill an old-fashioned glass with cubed ice. Add the sparkling water and Seedlip. Using a bar spoon, stir the ingredients together. Float the CBD oil drops on top and add the terpene enhancements (if using). Finally, garnish with your choice of accompaniments (if using) and enjoy!

GINGER RABBIT

Packed with nutrients, vitamins, and minerals, fresh carrot juice adds delicious flavors to drinks and can help improve your immune system, increase your metabolism, and help lower cholesterol. Carrot juice also mixes well with many other fruits, vegetables, roots, and herbs. Give this recipe a try when you're in need of some extra nutrients or anytime you're in the mood for an incredibly refreshing drink!

YIELD: 1 serving	**TARGET DOSE:** 8 mg CBD | 2 mg THC per drink (using Infused Ginger Simple Syrup, page 90) or your preferred dose (using a commercially made CBD or THC tincture of your choice, see note below)

EQUIPMENT
Muddler
Shaker tin
Fine-mesh strainer
Collins glass
Bar spoon
Reusable straw

INGREDIENTS
1 (1-inch or 2.5-cm) piece fresh ginger, peeled and sliced
2 ounces (60 ml) fresh-pressed apple juice
4 ounces (120 ml) fresh-pressed carrot juice
1½ ounces (45 ml) fresh squeezed lemon juice
½ ounce (15 ml) Infused Ginger Simple Syrup (page 90)
Ice
Splash ginger beer (I recommend Q brand, see note.)
Carrot greens, edible flowers, and a slice of lemon, for garnish

Muddle the ginger and apple juice at the bottom of a shaker tin. Muddle well to extract as much ginger flavor as possible. Add the carrot juice, lemon juice, and infused ginger simple syrup. Add ice, cover, then shake for 15 seconds or until very cold.

Using a fine-mesh strainer, separate the solids from the liquids over a Collins glass filled three-quarters with fresh ice. Top with a splash of ginger beer, give it a good stir with a bar spoon, then garnish with a sprig of carrot greens, edible flowers, and a slice of lemon. Enjoy with a reusable straw.

NOTE: *When making spirit-free mixed drinks, it's best to stick with healthier options and avoid extra sugar. Use fresh pressed juices over concentrates and source seasonal, fresh ingredients. And when it comes to ginger beer, the quality also matters. I recommend using Q ginger beer because of its extra carbonation and spicy but not overly sweet flavor. Avoid using mixers that contain high fructose corn syrup or a ton of added sugar, which can drastically change the drink's profile. If you don't have ginger simple syrup, substitute regular simple syrup, then add your favorite unflavored tincture (at your preferred dose) into the shaker before muddling. Follow the directions as written.*

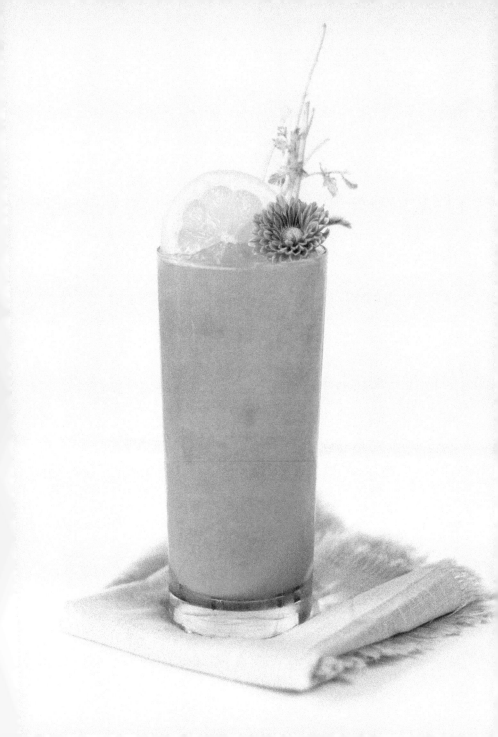

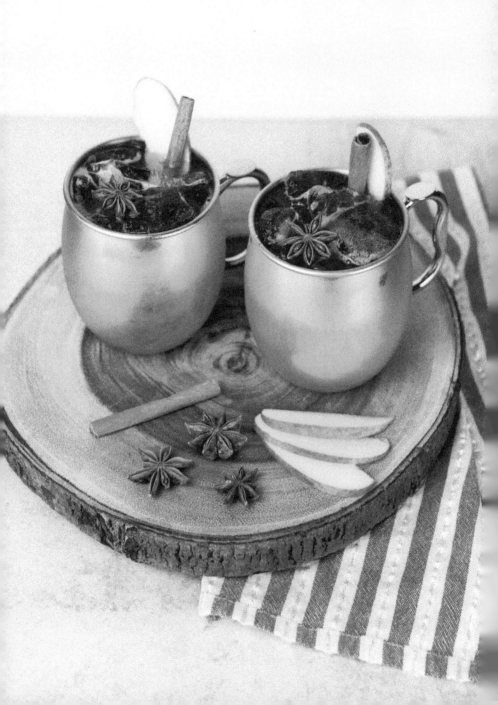

APPLE SPICE CBD MULE

Festive drinks with seasonal flavors are a must for the holidays. This gorgeous drink will keep the party vibes flowing, and it will also help your guests avoid that nasty holiday hangover. Combining the delicious flavors of apple cider, ginger beer, fresh squeezed lime juice, and Infused Cinnamon-Cardamom Simple Syrup (page 90), this recipe will become a holiday go-to.

YIELD: 1 serving	**TARGET DOSE:** 8 mg CBD ǀ 2 mg THC per drink (using Infused Cinnamon-Cardamom Simple Syrup, page 90) or your preferred dose (using commercially made CBD or THC tincture of your choice, see note below)

EQUIPMENT
Copper mug
Bar spoon

INGREDIENTS
3 ounces (90 ml) spiced apple cider (make your own for best flavor)
½ ounce (15 ml) Infused Cinnamon-Cardamom Simple Syrup (page 90)
½ ounce (15 ml) fresh squeezed lime juice
Ice to fill mug (cracked iced recommended but cubed ice works, too)
Ginger beer
Cinnamon stick, apple slice, and star anise, for garnish

Combine the spiced apple cider, infused simple syrup, and lime juice in a copper mug. Stir the ingredients well using a bar spoon. Fill the mug with ice, then top with ginger beer, slowly pouring until the mug is full. Give it a stir, then garnish with a cinnamon stick, an apple slice, and star of anise before serving.

HOW TO MAKE HOMEMADE SPICED APPLE CIDER

Add 8 apples of your choice (cut into quarters), ½ orange, 5 cinnamon sticks, 5 whole cardamom pods, 1 teaspoon whole allspice, 1 teaspoon whole cloves, 1 whole nutmeg, and ½ cup (100 g) packed golden brown sugar to a large stockpot. Cover with 1 to 2 inches (2.5 to 5 cm) of water, then bring to a boil. Stir, then cover the pot. Reduce the heat and simmer for 2 hours. Using a ladle, remove the orange and discard. Carefully mash the apples with a potato masher, then simmer the cider uncovered for another hour. Finally, strain the liquid through a fine-mesh strainer into a clean saucepan or pitcher. Enjoy hot or cold within one week.

SPIRIT-FREE MIXED DRINKS

NOTE

If you don't have the supplies to infuse CBD and THC into the cinnamon-cardamom simple syrup, simply substitute the non-infused version and add your favorite unflavored tincture (at your preferred dose) to the mixing glass. Then, proceed with the recipe.

FUZZY GINGER FIZZ

Playfully peachy, gingery, and spritzy, the Fuzzy Ginger Fizz is incredibly refreshing, yet tastes therapeutic due to the combination of ginger, peach, fresh squeezed lemon juice, and shrub. By muddling the ingredients, this drink is lively on the palate and glows with a peachy pink hue. To create the finest froth, make sure to dry shake first, then shake again with ice to cool the ingredients down. Top with ginger beer and watch the foam rise! Enjoy the fizzy flavors on your palate.

YIELD: **1** serving	**TARGET DOSE:** 6 mg CBD | 1.5 mg THC per drink (using Infused Ginger Peach Shrub, page 85) or your preferred dose (using commercially made CBD or THC tincture of your choice, see note below)

EQUIPMENT
Shaker tin
Muddler
Hawthorne strainer
Chilled old-fashioned glass

INGREDIENTS
¼ fresh, ripe large yellow peach, cut into pieces

1 (½-inch or 1-cm) piece fresh ginger, peeled and cut into pieces

1½ ounces (45 ml) Infused Ginger Peach Shrub (page 85)

1½ ounces (45 ml) fresh squeezed lemon juice

1 egg white

Ice

Ginger beer (I recommend Q brand, see note on page 130.)

Thin slice of peach and seasonal flowers, for garnish

In a shaker tin, add the peach, ginger, infused shrub, and lemon juice. Muddle the ingredients until the peach juices release. Use a Hawthorne strainer to separate and discard the solids. Pour the liquid back into the shaker.

Add the egg white, then cover and dry shake vigorously (no ice) for about 15 seconds. Add ice and shake again until very cold.

Strain the liquid into a chilled old-fashioned glass filled with fresh ice. Top with ginger beer, gently stir, then garnish with a thin slice of peach and seasonal flowers. Serve immediately.

NOTE *If you don't have the supplies to infuse CBD and THC into the ginger peach shrub, simply substitute for the non-infused version. Add the non-infused shrub and your favorite unflavored tincture (at your preferred dose) into the shaker tin before dry shaking, then follow the directions as written.*

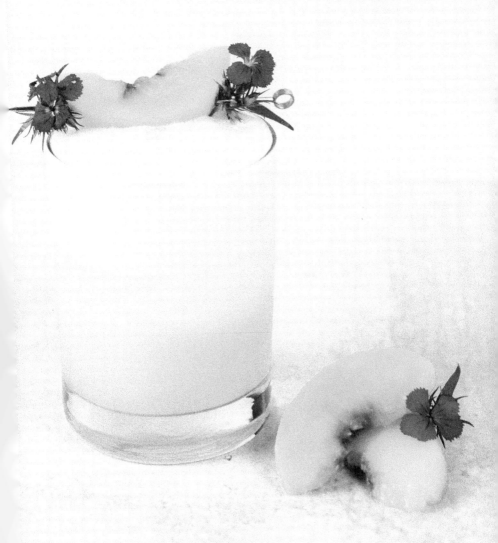

THE JOLLY CRANBERRY

There's no better time to enjoy a cheerful cranberry drink than during the holidays. Served in a chilled champagne flute and topped with all of the festive fixings, this is the perfect infused beverage for celebration. With a boost of citrus to keep spirits bright, put your mixology skills to the test and create your own cannabis-infused cranberry shrub. Top with sparkling apple cider to ring in the season's best flavors!

YIELD: 1 serving	**TARGET DOSE:** 3 mg CBD | < 1 mg THC per drink (using Infused Cranberry Shrub, see opposite) or your preferred dose (using commercially made CBD or THC tincture of your choice, see note below)

EQUIPMENT
Chilled champagne flute
Shaker tin
Fine-mesh strainer
Bar spoon

SUGARED RIM
1 orange or lemon slice
1 tablespoon (13 g) sugar

THE JOLLY CRANBERRY
1 ounce (30 ml) Infused
   Cranberry Shrub (see
   opposite)
¾ ounce (22 ml) fresh
   squeezed lemon juice
Ice
Chilled sparkling apple cider
Frozen cranberries and a
   rosemary sprig, for garnish

To create a sugared rim: Rim the top of a champagne flute with an orange slice, then dip the flute into the sugar.

To make The Jolly Cranberry: Combine the infused shrub and lemon juice in a shaker tin, add ice, cover, and shake until very cold. Using a fine-mesh strainer, strain the liquid into the champagne flute, then top with chilled sparkling apple cider. Carefully stir a few times with a bar spoon, then garnish with a few frozen cranberries for a frosty look and a rosemary sprig.

CANNABIS DRINKS

NOTE

If you don't have the supplies to infuse CBD and THC into the cranberry shrub, simply substitute the non-infused version. Add the non-infused shrub and your favorite unflavored tincture (at your preferred dose) into the shaker tin with lemon juice, shrub, and ice. Shake until cold, then follow the directions as written.

HOW TO MAKE INFUSED CRANBERRY SHRUB

YIELD: 2 cups (480 ml)

This time we'll be using the "hot process" to create a shrub. Using a small
saucepan, bring 10 ounces (280 g) fresh cranberries, 1½ cups (360 ml) water,
1 cup (200 g) sugar, 1 teaspoon orange zest, 2 tablespoons (30 ml) fresh
squeezed orange juice, 1 cinnamon stick, and ½ teaspoon allspice to a simmer,
continuously stirring. Reduce the heat to low, then cook until most of the
cranberries have burst. Using a fine-mesh strainer, separate the solids from the
liquids, then chill the syrup. Once cooled, add ½ cup plus 1 tablespoon (135 ml)
red wine vinegar and 1 ounce (30 ml) Infused Alcohol Tincture (pages 79 to 80)
or unflavored alcohol tincture of your choice. Whisk, then transfer to an airtight
swing bottle, and store in the refrigerator until further use. If you'd like to use
the leftover cranberry solids, I recommend blending them into a purée to use in
other recipes. Don't forget to remove the cinnamon stick before blending!

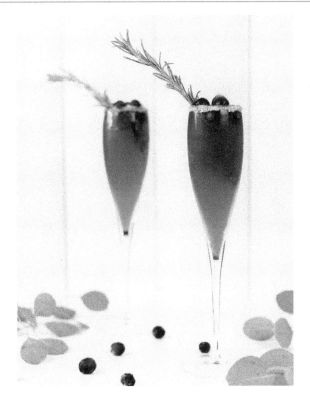

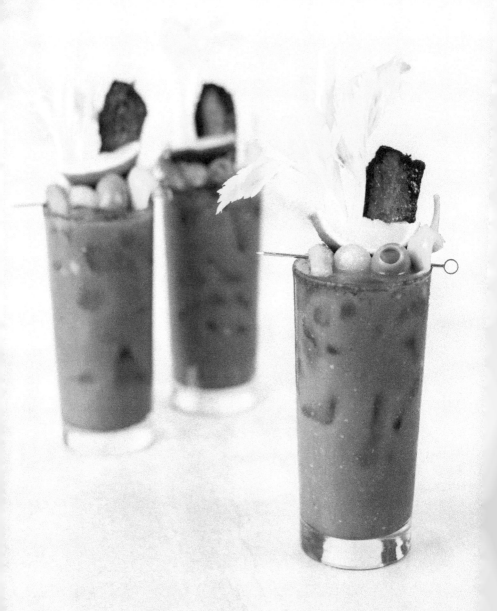

FEISTY MARY

Most often considered the ultimate brunch drink, every aspiring mixologist should know how to craft an out-of-this-world delicious Bloody Mary. When it comes to this popular tomato-based beverage, many variations will work, especially when creatively combining myriad savory and spicy ingredients. Here's my alcohol-free take on this cult-classic, the Feisty Mary. Handcrafted with my homemade infused Feisty Sauce and Infused Celery Bitters (page 83), I hope you're ready for some heat!

YIELD: **1** serving for drink and Feisty Sauce. 10 servings for bacon	**TARGET DOSE:** your preferred dose (using a commercially made CBD or THC tincture of your choice, see Feisty Sauce, page 140) + 2 mg CBD | < 1 mg THC per drink (using Infused Celery Bitters, page 83)

EQUIPMENT

Mixing bowl
Cooling rack
Baking sheet
Highball glass
Single-serve blender
One 4-ounce (120-ml)
    sterilized Mason jar
Boston shaker
Reusable straw

CANDIED BACON

¾ cup (113 g) golden brown
    sugar
1 tablespoon (7 g) paprika
½ teaspoon black pepper
1 (16-ounce, or 454-g) pack
    thick-cut bacon

Preheat the oven to 425°F (220°C, or gas mark 7). Place a cooling rack on top of a baking sheet.

To make the candied bacon: While the oven is heating, combine the golden brown sugar, paprika, and black pepper to taste in a mixing bowl. Stir together well. Coat each piece of bacon with the sugar mix. Add more brown sugar and spices if needed, then place on the cooling rack positioned on the baking sheet. This will ensure your bacon is extra crispy and candied to perfection. Bake for 15 to 20 minutes, checking in frequently to see if it's crispy to your liking. Continue to bake for 5 minutes if it needs some extra time. After the bacon is done cooking, remove from the oven, then let cool on the cooling rack.

(continued)

FEISTY SAUCE

¾ ounce (22 ml) fresh squeezed lemon juice

½ fresh serrano pepper (for more heat, add the full pepper)

CBD or THC tincture of your choice (at your preferred dose)

2 deli sliced peperoncini rings

1 teaspoon peperoncini juice

1 teaspoon green olive juice

1 teaspoon pickle juice

1 teaspoon freshly prepared horseradish

½ teaspoon fresh dill

⅛ teaspoon ground cinnamon

⅛ teaspoon celery salt

⅛ teaspoon ground cumin

⅛ teaspoon chili powder

⅛ teaspoon cayenne pepper

Dash black pepper

Dash red pepper flakes

Next, it's time to create the Feisty Sauce: Add all the ingredients to a single-serve blender and blend until smooth. Empty into a 4-ounce (120-ml) Mason jar and set aside.

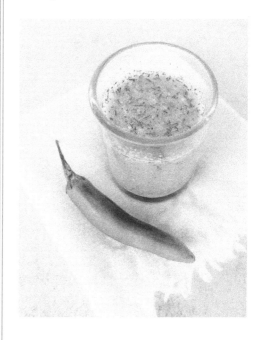

CHILE SALT RIM

1 lime wedge

1 teaspoon ancho chile powder or standard chile powder

2 teaspoons salt

FEISTY MARY

1½ ounces (45 ml) Feisty Sauce

7 ounces (210 ml) tomato juice

½ ounce (15 ml) fresh squeezed lime juice

2 dashes (12 to 16 drops or ¼ teaspoon) Infused Celery Bitters (page 83)

1 or 2 dashes Worcestershire sauce

Pinch salt

Ice

Candied bacon, celery, lime wedge, and your favorite pickled vegetables, for garnish

To make the chile salt rim: While the bacon is cooling, rim a highball glass with a lime wedge. On a small plate, stir together the chile powder and salt, then dip the glass rim into the chile salt to create a salted rim. Set aside.

To make the Feisty Mary: In Boston shaker, combine the Feisty Sauce, tomato juice, lime juice, infused bitters, Worcestershire sauce, and salt in one part of the shaker. To create the best consistency, you'll want to "roll" this Feisty Mary instead of shaking or stirring. To do so, add ice to the other part of the Boston shaker. Pour the liquid ingredients over the ice, then roll the liquid back and forth between both shakers about 5 or 6 times to mix the ingredients. Pour the liquid and ice into the salt-rimmed highball glass, then garnish with candied bacon, celery, lime wedge, and an array of pickled vegetables.

NOTE

To make more than one drink, prepare a big batch of the Feisty Sauce. Just be sure to use a jigger to measure the sauce and precisely dose. If you don't have the supplies to make the infused celery bitters, simply skip this step and follow the directions as written.

THE BOTANIST

Fresh from the garden, this delicious ensemble of fruits, vegetables, flowers, cannabis, and herbs would do any botanist proud! Enchanting with its green hue, creamy mouthfeel, and delicate flavor, this refreshing drink is guaranteed to delight the palate, highlighting a complex blend of aromas and flavors. The Botanist is a perfect option to serve during the springtime as plants begin to awaken. Quench your thirst while providing your body with a boost of plant-based nutrition and bliss.

YIELD: **1** serving	**TARGET DOSE:** 7.5 mg CBD | 2 mg THC per drink (using Infused Rich Simple Syrup, page 89) or your preferred dose (using commercially made CBD or THC tincture of your choice, see note below)

EQUIPMENT
Shaker tin
Muddler
Fine-mesh strainer
Chilled sour glass

INGREDIENTS
5 thick slices English cucumber, peeled and chopped
4 sugar snap peas, chopped
½ teaspoon chopped fresh tarragon
1½ ounces (45 ml) fresh squeezed lemon juice
2 ounces (60 ml) freshly brewed chamomile tea (room temperature or chilled)
½ teaspoon rosewater
½ ounce (15 ml) Infused Rich Simple Syrup (page 89)

1 egg white
Ice
Edible flowers and spring greens (or live pea tendrils, if you can find them), for garnish

In a shaker tin, combine the cucumber, sugar snap peas, fresh tarragon, lemon juice, chamomile tea, and rosewater. Muddle the ingredients together for 1 to 2 minutes to extract as much juice, color, and flavor as possible. Strain out the solids and pour the liquid back into the shaker. Discard the solids. Add the infused simple syrup and the egg white, then cover and dry shake (no ice) for 15 seconds. Add ice and shake again for 15 seconds, or until very cold.

Using a fine-mesh strainer, strain the liquid over a chilled sour glass. Shake the strainer to capture as much froth as possible. Garnish with edible flowers and spring greens or pea tendrils, then enjoy.

NOTE: *If you don't have the supplies to infuse the rich simple syrup, substitute the non-infused version and add your favorite unflavored tincture (at your preferred dose) to the shaker tin before dry shaking. Then, proceed with the recipe.*

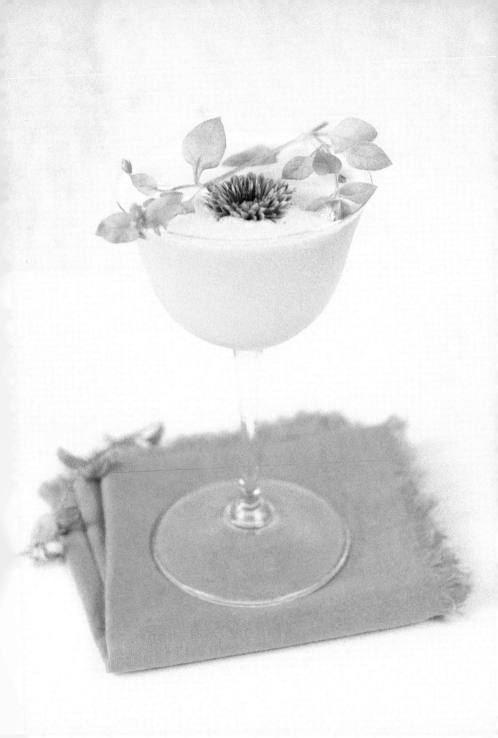

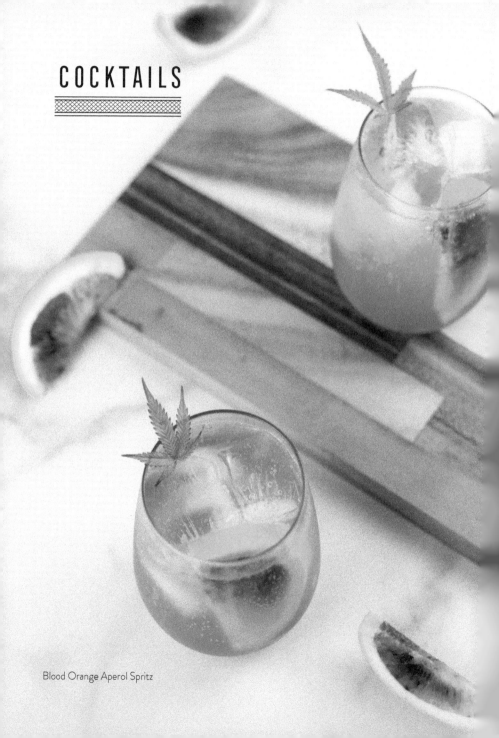

COCKTAILS

Blood Orange Aperol Spritz

BLOOD ORANGE
APEROL SPRITZ

When it comes to refreshing drinks, it doesn't get much better than an Aperol spritz. Unlike Campari, Aperol is lower in alcohol (11 percent ABV), and when mixed with prosecco and sparkling water, it's the perfect aperitif served during cocktail hour. Aperol is a fantastic companion for cannabis because it presents a botanical blend of herbs, roots, and citrus aromas and flavors. For a special winter twist, try adding blood oranges and a few dashes of Infused Citrus Spice Bitters (page 81) to microdose this classic European recipe.

YIELD: 1 serving	TARGET DOSE: between 2 mg CBD | < 1 mg THC per spritz (using Infused Citrus Spice Bitters, page 81) or your preferred dose (using commercially made CBD or THC alcohol tincture of your choice, see note below)

EQUIPMENT
Stemless wine glass
Jigger
Bar spoon

INGREDIENTS
Ice
½ ounce (15 ml) fresh squeezed blood orange juice, pulp removed
2 ounces (60 ml) Aperol
3 ounces (89 ml) dry prosecco
Club soda
2 dashes or ¼ teaspoon Infused Citrus Spice Bitters (page 81)
Blood orange slice, for garnish

Fill a wine glass about halfway full with ice. Add the blood orange juice, Aperol, and prosecco. Top the drink with your desired amount of club soda and add a dash or two of infused bitters. Using a bar spoon, gently stir the ingredients together, then add a slice of blood orange for garnish. Enjoy!

IMPORTANT: *As we've discussed, there are a few precautions you should take before mixing cannabis and hemp products with alcohol (refer to page 50). Remember that while CBD does not have the same intoxicating side effects as THC, the interactions between cannabidiol and alcohol is not thoroughly researched. It's best to proceed with caution and stick to the low side of the dosage range, which is reflected in the recipes found in this section. Start low, go slow.*

NOTE

If you don't have the supplies to infuse the citrus spice bitters at home, simply substitute your favorite bitters and unflavored tincture (at your preferred dose) and add to the wine glass before mixing. If you can source an alcohol-based tincture, this will blend seamlessly into the drink versus adding an oil.

SECRETS TO CRAFTING CANNABIS COCKTAILS

featuring Warren Bobrow, The Cocktail Whisperer,
author & cannabis alchemist

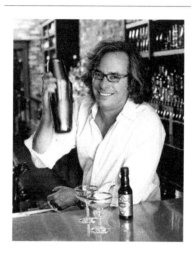

Warren Bobrow, aka The Cocktail Whisperer, is the author of six books on his own style of mixology including his celebrated release, Cannabis Cocktails, Mocktails, and Tonics. *He's a classically trained chef and bartender with hundreds of cocktail recipes to his name. Warren has written several articles for* Forbes, Saveur, Voda, Whole Foods-Dark Rye, Distiller, Beverage Media, DrinkUpNY, *and other international periodicals. Follow his cocktail adventures on Twitter @WarrenBobrow1 or Instagram @warrenbobrow.*

WARREN BOBROW: "Using cannabis in a cocktail doesn't change anything but the buzz! The cocktails are exactly the same. It's just the infused ingredients that add depth and balance.

When creating cannabis cocktails, I always stick to the principles of bartending, thus, no shaking a Manhattan or a gin martini. It's just not done, no matter what James Bond does! Another tip I like to recommend is to remember to use bitters, and I'm not just talking about Angostura. Bitter Truth, Fee Brothers, and Scrappy's all make worthy versions of bitters (or make your own). Each has its own charm and depth. With just one drop, bitters will make your cannabis or CBD cocktails sing!

One of the most important things when crafting cannabis cocktails is to start by sourcing quality ingredients: Craft spirits over the big market brands, not using spirits that are caramel-colored, or pad filtered, or sugar added. Haven't we had enough sugar already?! I also use the finest citrus fruits and, of course, the bitters component. I never skimp. Drinks will always be better because of the fine ingredients you use from the start.

Another tip is to look for bright and lively flavors to balance against the deeper aromatics of the cannabis. For example, I love to roast fruits to the caramelization phase and cool and juice them to reveal their secrets! Should you not be able to find great citrus, I suggest using a pure fruit syrup from Massachusetts named Fruitations. This product is brilliant!

When searching for cannabis strains to work with, Mango Trainwreck is one of my favorites. I especially like this strain in nanotechnology with terpenes (the stuff that smells like weed!). I also love the strain, Dr. Grinspoon, from an ultra-high-quality craft grower named Excelsior Extracts. Amazing with mezcal!

If you're a beginner using cannabis to make infusions at home and forget to decarboxylate—woes be! Nothing will happen. You'll never get "high" if you don't activate your flower. To a certain extent, the same holds true for CBD. If you're looking for a buzz, good luck with that. There's only trace amounts of THC in hemp—any "stoned" feelings you get are purely imaginary. Remember, CBD will not make you high!

Here's an infused cocktail recipe I call Gin & Bedeviled. Enjoy."

GIN & BEDEVILED

YIELD: 2 servings

TARGET DOSE: Your preferred dose

EQUIPMENT
Baking sheet
Boston shaker
2 coupe glasses

INGREDIENTS
½ orange
Ice
4 ounces (120 ml) botanical gin (like Hendrick's)
¼ ounce (7 ml) simple syrup
Fee Brothers West Indian Orange Bitters
Fee Brothers Lemon Bitters
Cannabis-infused bitters of your choice or Infused Citrus Spice Bitters (page 81)
1 ounce (30 ml) Q Club Soda
Orange zest, flamed

Prepare the oven-roasted juice. Preheat the oven to 275°F (140°C, or gas mark 1). Place the orange half in a small baking dish and roast for 1 hour. Cool and juice, then set aside.

Next, fill a Boston shaker with ice to three-quarters full. Add 2 ounces (30 ml) of oven-roasted orange juice, the gin, and the simple syrup. Cap and shake hard for 20 seconds. Pour into two coupe glasses. Dot with the bitters. Dot with the cannabis-infused bitters, then add a splash of club soda for lift. Garnish with a flamed orange zest.

LAID-BACK MANHATTAN

If you're a rye lover, the Manhattan might top your list when it comes to the most delicious cocktail recipes. Typically offering a 2:1 ratio of rye whiskey to sweet vermouth, this drink dates back to the 1880s after first appearing at New York City's Manhattan Club, so the legend goes. Giving the Manhattan a laid-back twist, add a few dashes of Infused Citrus Spice Bitters (page 81) to mildly elevate this time-honored classic.

YIELD: **1** serving	**TARGET DOSE:** 2 mg CBD | < 1 mg THC per drink (using Infused Citrus Spice Bitters, page 81) or your preferred dose (using commercially made CBD or THC alcohol tincture of your choice, see note below)

EQUIPMENT
Chilled Nick & Nora or
   martini glass
Mixing glass
Bar spoon

INGREDIENTS
Ice
2 ounces (60 ml) rye
   whiskey
1 ounce (30 ml) sweet
   vermouth
2 dashes or ¼ teaspoon
   Infused Citrus Spice
   Bitters (page 81)
1 maraschino cherry

Chill the glass by placing it in the freezer. While the glass is chilling, fill a mixing glass halfway with ice and add the rye whiskey, sweet vermouth, and infused bitters. Stir the mixture for about 15 seconds or until the liquid is very cold. Strain into the chilled glass, then add a maraschino cherry before serving.

COCKTAILS

NOTE

If you don't have the supplies to infuse the citrus spice bitters at home, simply substitute 1 or 2 dashes of aromatic bitters and your favorite un-flavored alcohol tincture (not oil!) at your preferred dose, then add both ingredients to the mixing glass before stirring.

SPICY MELON MARGARITA

This mouthwatering cannabis-infused melon margarita is the perfect
infused cocktail to serve during a summer barbecue. Made with fresh
watermelon juice, lime juice, Infused Rich Simple Syrup (page 89),
jalapeño chiles, and a splash of mezcal, tequila blanco, and Aperol, this
refreshing drink is served with a kick from the chile rim.

YIELD: **1** serving	**TARGET DOSE:** 7.5 mg CBD | 2 mg THC per drink (using Infused Rich Simple Syrup, page 89) or your preferred dose (using commercially made CBD or THC tincture of your choice, see note below)

EQUIPMENT
Blender or food processor
Fine-mesh strainer
One 8-ounce (240-ml)
   sterilized Mason jar
Saucer
Citrus juicer
Old-fashioned glass
Shaker tin
Jigger
Hawthorne strainer

WATERMELON JUICE
½ small seedless watermelon

CHILE SALT RIM
1 tablespoon (9 g) salt
¼ teaspoon ancho chile
   powder or standard chili
   powder
1 lime wedge

SPICY MELON MARGARITA
1¼ ounce (38 ml) fresh
   squeezed lime juice
½ ounce (15 ml) Infused
   Rich Simple Syrup
   (page 89)

½ ounce (15 ml) tequila blanco
½ ounce (15 ml) mezcal
½ teaspoon Aperol
1 small jalapeño pepper, sliced into rounds (set
   1 round aside for garnish)
Ice
Lime round, for garnish (optional)

To make the watermelon juice: Place the
watermelon flesh into a blender or food processor.
Purée for 1 minute or until the watermelon chunks
turn into juice. Using a fine-mesh strainer, separate
the pulp from the juice over an 8-ounce (240-ml)
Mason jar. Discard the pulp and set the jar aside.

To create the chili rim: Combine the salt and chile
powder in a shallow saucer. Rim the glass with a
lime wedge, then dip the glass into the salt mixture
creating the chile rim. If you have Tajín on hand,
this works great, too!

To make the Spicy Melon Margarita: Add all the
ingredients into a shaker tin, including 3 ounces
(90 ml) of watermelon juice and the jalapeños.
Add ice, cover, then shake for 25 seconds. Fine
strain into an old-fashioned glass filled with fresh
ice. Garnish with jalapeño rounds or a lime wheel.

If you don't have the supplies to infuse the rich simple syrup at home, simply substitute regular simple syrup and add your favorite unflavored tincture (at your preferred dose) into the shaker tin, then follow the directions as written.

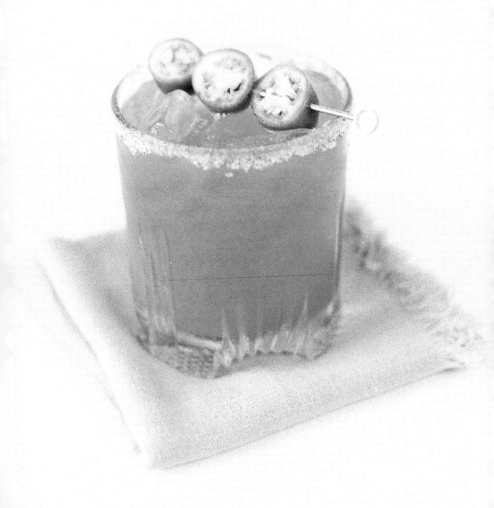

INFUSING SEASONAL
SPIRIT-FREE COCKTAILS

featuring Rachel Burkons of Altered Plates

Rachel Burkons is the co-founder of Los Angeles–based hospitality company, Altered Plates. After spending more than a decade in the wine and spirits industry as the cannabis editor for national publication The Clever Root, *and the VP/Associate Publisher for sister publications* The Tasting Panel *and* The SOMM Journal, *Rachel is an expert mixologist and one of the leading voices in exploring the connection between food, drinks, and cannabis. With close ties to top chefs, mixologists, and sommelier tastemakers across the country, she is also a leading educator and hospitality consultant that specializes in the cannabis space. For more cannabis cocktail and hospitality tips, follow Rachel @smokesipsavor or visit her website at RachelBurkons.com.*

RACHEL BURKONS: "While seasonality is an important consideration when crafting cocktails or spirit-free drinks all year long, there's something special about springtime. With so many bright, blooming flowers and fruits, beautiful aromas wafting through the air, and vibrant colors exploding everywhere, springtime is a true delight for the senses. When it comes to translating all of that magic to the glass, look for those same bright colors, sweet floral notes, and bold aromatics. Spring cocktails should be fresh and vibrant, and with so many wonderful ingredients coming into season this time of year, you can let what's local and fresh guide you. Late winter/early spring is also all about citrus fruits, and with limes in abundance this time of year, you can create beautiful drinks bursting with both flavor and spring's signature color—green!

To celebrate spring, feel illuminated inside and out with The Limelight. Tapping into lime's natural limonene-rich properties, this mood-enhancing infused beverage is incredibly thirst-quenching. Lime juice is also an excellent source of vitamin C and potassium, providing immune-boosting effects. Enjoy this recipe as an aperitif or digestif: It's light, refreshing, and incredibly delicious!"

THE LIMELIGHT

YIELD: **1** serving

TARGET DOSE: your preferred dose (using a commercially made CBD or THC tincture of your choice)

EQUIPMENT
Shaker tin
Hawthorn strainer
Champagne flute

INGREDIENTS
1½ ounces (45 ml) fresh squeezed lime juice
1½ ounces (45 ml) lime syrup
CBD or THC tincture of your choice (at your preferred dose)
Ice
Sparkling mineral water
1 key lime wheel or finger lime pearls (optional)

Combine the lime juice, lime syrup, and infused tincture of your choice in a shaker tin, over ice. Place the lid on the tin and shake for 10 seconds. Strain, pouring the liquid into a champagne flute. Top with your choice of sparkling mineral water. Garnish with a key lime wheel or with lime pearls (if using) as floating "bubbles."

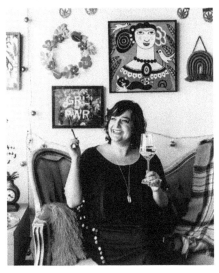

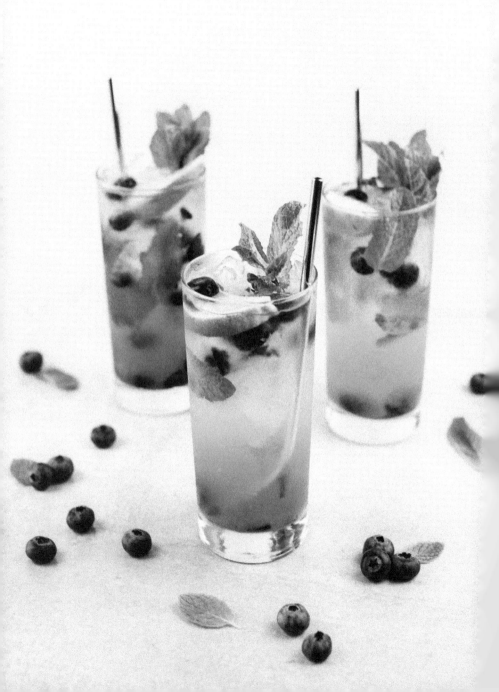

BLUE DREAM BERRY MOJITO

The mojito is a classic drink that typically consists of five ingredients: mint, lime, simple syrup, club soda, and rum. Add blueberries and cannabis, even better! This fizzy, thirst-quenching infused blueberry mojito is easy to make, plus Instagram-worthy with it's beautiful blue and purple hue. Perfect for enjoying during those lazy weekend afternoons, treat your palate to this refreshing aperitif before a meal.

YIELD: 1 serving	**TARGET DOSE:** 7.5 mg CBD | 2 mg THC per drink (using Infused Rich Simple Syrup, page 89) or your preferred dose (using commercially made CBD or THC tincture of your choice, see note below)

EQUIPMENT
Highball glass
Muddler
Bar spoon

INGREDIENTS
¾ ounce (22 ml) fresh squeezed lime juice
8 fresh mint leaves, plus more leaves for the glass
2 lime wedges
⅓ cup (50 g) fresh blueberries, plus more whole blueberries for the glass
½ ounce (15 ml) Infused Rich Simple Syrup (page 89)
Cracked ice
1½ ounces (45 ml) white rum

Club soda
Dash of Angostura bitters (optional)
Fresh mint sprig, lime wedge, and blueberries, for garnish

In a highball glass, add the lime juice. Smack the mint leaves, then add them to the glass along with the lime wedges and blueberries. Using a muddler, gently muddle the ingredients to release the mint oils and juices. Add the infused simple syrup, then muddle again (be careful not to tear the mint leaves or over muddle!). Fill the glass to the top with cracked ice, layering in a few fresh blueberries and mint leaves. Add as much ice as possible. Add the rum, then top with club soda and a dash of Angostura bitters. Stir well with a bar spoon. Garnish with a mint sprig (make sure to smack the leaves!), a lime wedge, and fresh blueberries before serving.

NOTE ‖ *If you don't have the supplies to infuse the rich simple syrup at home, simply substitute regular rich simple syrup and add your favorite unflavored tincture (at your preferred dose) into the highball glass before muddling, then follow the directions as written.*

155

COCKTAILS

STRAWBERRY-RHUBARB SHRUB SODA

Both sweet and tart with a boost of botanicals, this strawberry-rhubarb shrub soda is so light and refreshing, you'll want to drink two! Combining a symphony of flavors, this drink blends sweet strawberry with citrus and rhubarb notes that cleanse the palate. The vodka's subtle profile is a perfect match for this shrub cocktail. Enjoy this thirst-quenching beverage on a warm spring or summer day.

YIELD: **1** serving	**TARGET DOSE:** 4 mg CBD | 1 mg THC per drink (using Infused Strawberry Lime Shrub, page 86) or your preferred dose (using commercially made CBD or THC tincture of your choice, see note below)

EQUIPMENT
Shaker tin
Muddler
Jigger
Hawthorne strainer
Old-fashioned glass
Bar spoon

INGREDIENTS
5 strawberries, cut in half
¾ ounce (22 ml) fresh squeezed lemon juice
1 ounce (30 ml) Infused Strawberry Lime Shrub (page 86)
¾ ounce (22 ml) rhubarb liqueur
¾ ounce (22 ml) premium vodka
Ice

Club soda
Slice of strawberry, a lime wheel, and edible flowers, for garnish

In a shaker tin, muddle the strawberries until they release their juices. Add the lemon juice, shrub, rhubarb liqueur, vodka, and ice. Cover and shake for 15 seconds or until very cold. Strain into an old-fashioned glass filled with fresh ice. Top with club soda and give the drink a few good stirs using a bar spoon. Garnish with a slice of strawberry, lime wheel, and edible flowers.

NOTE

If you don't have the supplies to infuse CBD and THC into the strawberry lime shrub, simply use a non-infused version, then add your favorite unflavored tincture (at your preferred dose) into the shaker tin, then follow the directions as written.

CRAFTING CANNABIS COCKTAILS INSPIRED BY THE SENSES

featuring Tarita Noronha, cannabis mixologist & creator of Cannabixology

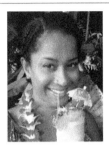

Since the early 2000s, Tarita has enjoyed a successful career in the adult beverage world. She spent many years perfecting her mixing craft in the dining scenes of New York City, San Francisco, and Las Vegas, and eventually settling in Los Angeles. From her experience in global Michelin-starred restaurants to her dedication in continued wine and spirits education, she elevated her career when she became the Spirits Specialist of a highly crafted portfolio for the state of California and Nevada. All the while, cannabis medical use was changing, and recreational use was becoming a reality. Tarita saw the need to use her expertise for the good of the movement! She wanted to use mixology as a crossover point between both worlds and wanted to continue to educate, advocate, and work to remove the stigma of cannabis through delicious and approachable consumption. Follow Tarita's cannabis journey, plus discover her latest recipes and tips @cannabixology or visit www.cannabixology.com.

TARITA NORONHA: "So much of cocktail creation is playing with flavors and ingredients that inspire your senses. I love to mix ingredients that invoke feelings of nostalgia. My approach to cocktail creation is the same as when I cook. We're not reinventing the wheel; we're just trying to polish it with some love and our own special spice.

Many CBD and THC tinctures available on the market are already mixed with a carrier oil, and it can help make a cocktail with fat-soluble ingredients. But, if you're lucky to find a water-soluble tincture, then a gold star for you! Either way, cannabinoids are absorbed more efficiently into your body through a base such as coconut milk. A well-known cocktail inspiration comes to mind. It's tropical but oh so sinfully delightful, the Piña Colada!

My guilt-free variation utilizes turmeric and ginger syrup. These flavors bring me back to my Indian roots. Ancient cultures have long been singing praises for these spices' healing attributes. The turmeric and ginger colada will be a party favorite, not too sweet, perfectly spiced with earthy undertones. Let's call it, the Mellow Yellow. Cannabis cocktails could and should easily share a place at the party, but the most important part is dosing. I believe 15 milligrams of CBD is a good amount on average, but just remember it's an average for a reason. When it comes to THC, start low and go slow. And for the rest of the ingredients, never compromise on quality and you'll make healthy taste great!

This spin on the tropical classic is a delicious earthy, spiced anti-inflammatory, anti-nausea, Ayurvedic vacation to the Far East. Shake well and prosper."

HOW TO MAKE GINGERROOT & TURMERIC SYRUP

1 cup (150 g) light brown cane sugar

1 cup (235 ml) filtered water

½ cup (96 g) peeled and thinly sliced fresh ginger

½ cup (50 g) peeled and chopped fresh turmeric (if using dried powder version 1 teaspoon)

Pinch black pepper

Over very low temperature, simmer all the ingredients for at least 1 hour. Take off heat and let cool. Continue to steep 4 to 8 hours. Strain with cheesecloth and keep in the refrigerator for up to 1 week.

MELLOW YELLOW

YIELD: **1** serving

TARGET DOSE: 15 milligrams CBD or 5 to 10 milligrams THC (using your choice of lab-tested cannabis oil or a water-soluble tincture)

EQUIPMENT
Tiki mug or Collins glass
Bar shaker set
Bar spoon
Hawthorne strainer
Mini umbrella

INGREDIENTS
Crushed ice

Lime wheel

3½ ounces (105 ml) coconut milk

1 ounce (30 ml) fresh squeezed lime juice

¾ ounce (22 ml) fresh Gingerroot & Turmeric Syrup (see recipe box opposite)

CBD or THC tincture of your choice

Club soda

Fresh mint leaves, for garnish

Prepare a tiki mug or a Collins glass by filling with crushed ice and laying the lime wheel inside as your garnish. Set aside.

In the shaker tin, combine the coconut milk, lime juice, syrup, and CBD or THC tincture. Cover and dry shake (no ice) to emulsify the oil-based tincture into the mix.

Once mixed well, add ice and shake again to chill. Strain over the fresh crushed ice in the glass. Top with club soda, give a final light stir, and garnish with mint leaves. Serve with a mini umbrella.

159

COCKTAILS

N O T E

To mix this as an alcoholic cocktail, I suggest 1½ ounces (45 ml) of light rum, vodka, or whiskey. If you want to make it nonalcoholic, you have that option as well. Remember, if you add alcohol and are mixing with THC, adjust the dosage down to play it safe.

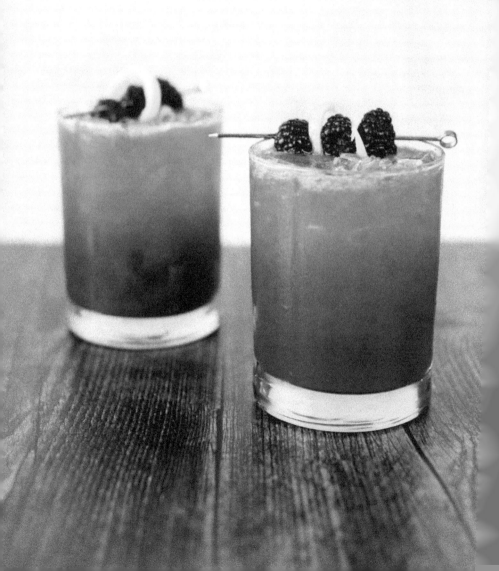

BLACKBERRY GINGER BRAMBLE

Originating in London in the 1980s, the Bramble traditionally incorporates dry gin, lemon juice, simple syrup, crème de mûre (a blackberry liquor), and crushed ice. As an old classic, here's a fun and refreshing cannabis-infused blackberry ginger Bramble you can try at home. Rather than using blackberry liqueur, try adding fresh blackberries, then muddle with your ingredients including infused ginger simple syrup. Add a splash of ginger beer and a dash of bitters for an extra kick of flavor!

YIELD: 1 serving	**TARGET DOSE:** 12 mg CBD | 3 mg THC per drink (using Infused Ginger Simple Syrup, page 90) or your preferred dose (using commercially made CBD or THC tincture of your choice, see note below)

EQUIPMENT
Shaker tin
Muddler
Old-fashioned glass
Hawthorne strainer
Fine-mesh strainer

INGREDIENTS
⅓ cup (43 g) fresh blackberries
1¼ ounces (38 ml) fresh squeezed lemon juice
¾ ounce (22 ml) dry gin
¾ ounce (22 ml) Infused Ginger Simple Syrup (page 90)
Cracked ice

Ginger beer (I recommend Q brand, see page 130.)
Dash Angostura bitters
Blackberries and a lemon twist, for garnish

In a shaker tin, muddle the blackberries with the lemon juice until the berries release their juices. Add the gin and infused simple syrup, then add ice. Cover and shake for 10 to 15 seconds. Fill an old-fashioned glass with fresh cracked ice. Place a Hawthorne strainer on the top of the shaker tin, then strain the liquid through a fine-mesh strainer over the old-fashioned glass to remove the seeds. Top with a splash of ginger beer and a dash of bitters. Give the drink a stir, then garnish with blackberries and a lemon twist.

NOTE

If you don't have the supplies to make infused ginger simple syrup, simply use non-infused simple syrup, add your favorite unflavored tincture (at your preferred dose) into the shaker tin, then follow the directions as written.

SPRING QUEEN

All hail the Spring Queen! This deliciously refreshing cannabis cocktail excites the palate with blissful notes of cucumber and citrus followed by a hint of elderflower. As a perfect aperitif to serve on a warm spring evening, dress up this drink with a crown of cucumber and seasonal flowers.

SERVINGS: **1**	**TARGET DOSE:** 4 mg CBD | 1 mg THC per drink (using Infused Rich Simple Syrup, page 89) or your preferred dose (using commercially made CBD or THC tincture of your choice, see note below)

EQUIPMENT
Shaker tin
Muddler
Fine-mesh strainer
Old-fashioned glass
Bar spoon

INGREDIENTS
4 thick slices English cucumber, cut into quarters
1¾ ounces (52 ml) fresh squeezed lime juice
¼ ounce (7.5 ml) Infused Rich Simple Syrup (page 89)
1½ ounces (45 ml) botanical gin (see note)
¾ ounce (22 ml) elderflower liqueur (see note)
Ice
Club soda
Cucumber ribbon and seasonal flower crown, for garnish

In a shaker tin, combine the cucumber, lime juice, and infused simple syrup. Muddle the ingredients to extract the cucumber's aromas and flavors. Add the gin, elderflower liqueur, and ice. Cover and shake for 15 seconds or until very cold. Fine strain into an old-fashioned glass filled with fresh ice. Add a splash of club soda and stir using a bar spoon. Garnish with a cucumber ribbon and seasonal flower crown.

NOTE: *For this recipe, I recommend using a botanical gin such as Hendrick's Gin and St. Germain Elderflower Liqueur for the best flavor. If you don't have the supplies to infuse the rich simple syrup at home, simply substitute regular rich simple syrup. Then, add your favorite unflavored CBD or THC tincture (at your preferred dose) into the shaker tin, then shake with the other ingredients. Follow the directions as written and enjoy!*

CANNABIS DRINKS

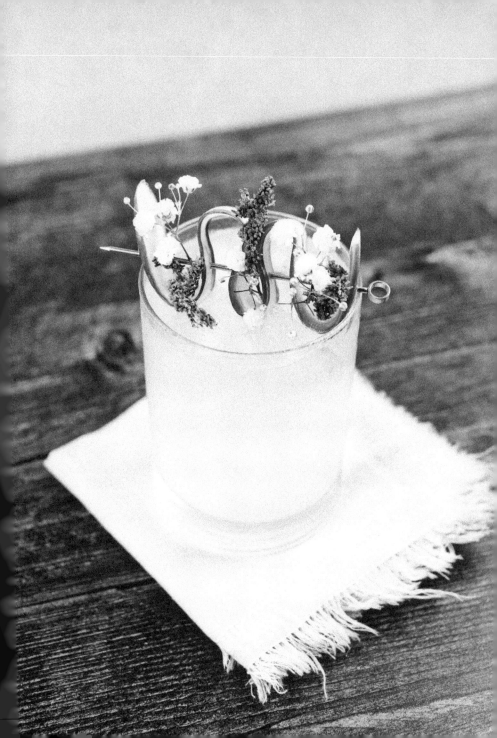

PAPAYA PISCO SOUR

If you've ever been to Peru or a Peruvian restaurant, it's hard to ignore the delicious pisco sour. This classic South American drink is creamy, yet bright with acidity and oh so refreshing! Give this Peruvian classic a tropical makeover; instead of adding traditional simple syrup, mix in Papaya Lime Syrup (page 165) for an extra special orange glow.

YIELD: 1 serving	TARGET DOSE: 4.5 mg CBD | 1.5 mg THC per drink (using Infused Sour Mix, page 93) or your preferred dose (using commercially made CBD or THC tincture of your choice, see note below)

EQUIPMENT
Chilled sour glass
Mixing bowls
Shaker tin
Hawthorne strainer

INGREDIENTS
1½ ounces (45 ml) pisco
1½ ounces (45 ml) Infused
    Sour Mix (page 93)
½ ounce (15 ml) fresh
    squeezed lime juice,
    pulp removed
1 ounce (30 ml) Papaya Lime
    Syrup (opposite)
1 egg white
Ice
Angostura bitters

Chill a sour glass by placing it in the freezer. While the glass is chilling, mix the pisco, infused sour mix, lime juice, papaya lime syrup, and egg white in a cocktail shaker. Cover and dry shake (no ice) for 10 seconds. Add ice, cover, and shake vigorously until very cold, creating as much froth as possible. Strain into the chilled sour glass and dot the foam with Angostura bitters before serving.

CANNABIS DRINKS

NOTE

If you don't have the supplies to infuse the sour mix, simply substitute the non-infused version and add your favorite unflavored tincture (at your preferred dose) to the shaker tin before dry shaking. Then, proceed with the recipe.

HOW TO MAKE PAPAYA LIME SYRUP

2 organic limes

¼ ripe medium papaya, cut into cubes (about 1½ cups, or 210 g)

½ cup (100 g) sugar

Using a zester, zest the limes over a mixing bowl. Combine the lime zest with the papaya and sugar. Stir together until the sugar coats the papaya completely. Cover the bowl with plastic wrap and store in the refrigerator overnight to macerate. The next day, give the mixture a good stir, then use a strainer to separate the newly formed syrup from the papaya solids over a mixing bowl. Discard the solids. Empty into a 4-ounce (120-ml) Mason jar and store in the refrigerator until you're ready to use. For best results and for the freshest flavor, use within one week.

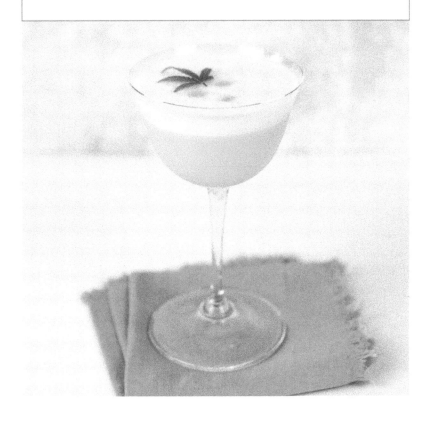

TOASTY TODDY

When it's chilly outside, nothing seems to warm the body quite like a Hot Toddy. If you're new to warm cocktails, this drink makes the perfect introduction, especially after a long day on the ski slopes or if you're battling a cold. Meet the Toasty Toddy. Incorporating toasted spices, spiced rum, Full-Spectrum Infused Honey (page 91), fresh squeezed lemon juice, hot water, and array of spiced garnishes, toast yourself up with this heartwarming cannabis cocktail on a cold winter's day.

YIELD: **1** serving	**TARGET DOSE:** 15 mg CBD | 2 mg THC per drink (using Full-Spectrum Infused Honey, page 91) or your preferred dose (using commercially made CBD or THC alcohol tincture of your choice, see note below)

EQUIPMENT
Measuring spoons
Small sauté pan or skillet
Measuring cup
Small saucepan
Fine-mesh strainer
Warmed cocktail coffee glass
  or glass of your choice
Measuring spoon
Bar spoon

INGREDIENTS
½ teaspoon whole cloves
1 cinnamon stick
4 semi-cracked cardamom
  pods
1 cup (240 ml) hot water
1½ ounces (45 ml) spiced
  rum (or whiskey if you
  prefer)
1 tablespoon (21 g) Full-
  Spectrum Infused
  Honey (page 91)

2 teaspoons fresh squeezed lemon juice
Dash Angostura bitters
Winter spices and a lemon round, for garnish

Begin by toasting the spices. Place the whole cloves, cinnamon stick, and whole cardamom pods in a small sauté pan over medium heat. Continue to shake the pan or use a spatula to move the spices around to keep them from burning. Remove from the heat once the spices become fragrant and set aside.

Add the water to a small saucepan and bring to a boil. Add the toasted spices, then reduce to a simmer for 10 minutes to take on the spiced flavors. Remove from the heat. Using a fine-mesh strainer, separate the solids from the liquid and empty the spiced water into a warmed cocktail coffee glass. Add the spiced rum, infused honey, and lemon juice to taste, then give the mixture a couple of stirs using a bar spoon until the honey fully dissolves. Garnish with winter spices and a lemon round before serving.

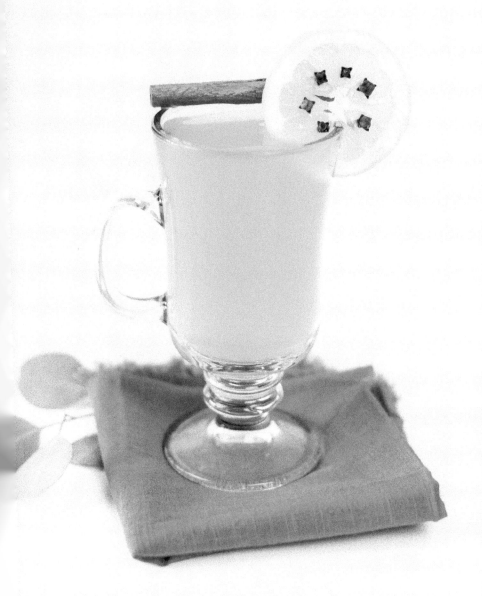

Aldin, Ben. "What Is Terpinolene and What Does This Cannabis Terpene Do?" *Leafly*. September 2018.

Amann. K., et al. *Drinking Like Ladies*. Beverly, MA: Quarto Publishing Group, 2018.

Bennett, P. "What Is Ocimene and What Does This Cannabis Terpene Do?" *Leafly*. December 2018.

Bobrow, Warren. *Cannabis Cocktails, Mocktails & Tonics*. Beverly, MA: Quarto Publishing Group USA Inc, 2016.

Boggs, D. L., et al. "Clinical and Preclinical Evidence for Functional Interactions of Cannabidiol and Δ9-Tetrahydrocannabinol." *Neuropsychopharmacology*. January 2018.

Booth, J. K., et al. "Terpene Synthases from *Cannabis sativa*." *PLOS One*. March 2017.

Boudinot, Jennifer. "Cocktails with Chronic: How to Infuse Liquor with Weed." *Paste Magazine*. February 6, 2017.

Bridgeman, M. B. "Medicinal Cannabis: History, Pharmacology, and Implications for the Acute Care Setting." *Pharmacy & Therapeutics*. March 2017.

Bruni, N., et al. "Cannabinoid Delivery Systems for Pain and Inflammation Treatment." *Molecules*. October 2018.

Budiaman, Will. *Handcrafted Bitters*. Berkeley, CA: Rockridge Press, 2015.

Builder, M. "The Types of Cocktail Glasses You Actually Need, According to Bartenders." *New York Magazine*. April 2018.

Chung T., R. A. Harris. "Cannabis and Alcohol: From Basic Science to Public Policy." *Alcoholism: Clinical and Experimental Research*. July 2, 2019.

Dao, Dan Q. "CBD Cocktails: What They Are and Why They're Taking Over Bar Menus Everywhere." *Food & Wine Magazine*. October 1, 2018.

Devitt-Lee, A. "CBD-Drug Interactions: Role of Cytochrome P450." *Project CBD*. September 8, 2015.

De Gregorio, D., et al. "Cannabidiol Modulates Serotonergic Transmission and Reverses Both Allodynia and Anxiety-Like Behavior in a Model of Neuropathic Pain." *PAIN*. January 2019.

De Ternay, J., M. Naassila, et al. "Therapeutic Prospects of Cannabidiol for Alcohol Use Disorder and Alcohol-Related Damages on the Liver and the Brain." *Frontiers in Pharmacology*. May 31, 2019.

Dietsch, M. *Shrubs*. New York, NY: The Countryman Press, 2016.

Evans. J. *The Ultimate Guide to CBD: Explore the World of Cannabidiol*. Beverly, MA: Quarto Publishing Group, 2018

Fernández-Ruiz, et al. "Cannabidiol for neurodegenerative Disorders: Important New Clinical Applications for This Phytocannabinoid?" *British Journal of Clinical Pharmacology*. May 25, 2012.

Gallily, R., et al. "The Anti-Inflammatory Properties of Terpenoids from Cannabis." *Cannabis Cannabinoid Research*. December 2018.

Goldleaf Ltd. *The Cooking Journal: A Cannabis Culinary Companion*. Fairfield, OH: Goldleaf Ltd., 2018.

Hodgins, P. "Mixology 101: Here Are 10 Reminders about What Makes a Winning Drink." *Good Liberations/The Orange County Register*. May 2015.

Huestis, M. A., et al. "Cannabidiol Adverse Effects and Toxicity." *Current Neuropharmacology*. June 3, 2019.

June-Wells, Mark, Ph.D. "Your Guide to Ethanol Extraction." *Cannabis Business Times*. July 11, 2018.

CANNABIS DRINKS

Korkidis, John. "Fat-Washed Cannabis-Infused Alcohol." *Chron Vivant*. December 29, 2017.

Lee, Martin A. "Cannabis Dosing 101." *Project CBD*. May 2018.

Lee, Martin A. "Terpenes and the 'Entourage Effect'" *Project CBD*.

Leinow, L. J. Birnbaum. *CBD: A Patient's Guide to Medical Cannabis*. Berkeley, CA: North Atlantic Books, 2017.

Magner, Erin. "What Really Happens When You Mix CBD and Alcohol." *Well Good*. September 28, 2019.

Mark, Kendra. "How Sunflower Lecithin May Help CBD Work Better and Faster." *2RiseNatural*. June 26, 2017.

Millar, S. A., et al. "A Systematic Review on the Pharmacokinetics of Cannabidiol in Humans." *Frontiers in Pharmacology*. November 26, 2018.

Millar, S. A., et al. "A Systematic Review of Cannabidiol Dosing in Clinical Populations." *British Journal of Clinical Pharmacology*. June 20, 2019.

Modesto Nascimento Menezes P., et al. "Cannabis and Cannabinoids on Treatment of Inflammation: A Patent Review." *Recent Patents on Biotechnology*. June 18, 2019.

Mudge E. M., et al. "The Terroir of Cannabis: Terpene Metabolomics as a Tool to Understand *Cannabis sativa* Selections." *Planta Medica*. July 2019.

Murrieta, E. "Will Infused Drinks Change How We Consume Cannabis?" *San Francisco Chronicle*. October 2019.

Nona, C. N., C. S. Hendershot, and B. Le Foll. "Effects of Cannabidiol on Alcohol-related Outcomes: A Review of Preclinical and Human Research." *Experimental and Clinical Psychopharmacology*. May 23, 2019.

Nuutinen, T., et al. "Medicinal Properties of Terpenes Found in *Cannabis sativa* and *Humulus lupulus*." *European Journal of Medicinal Chemistry*. 2018.

Owram, Kristine. "Scientists Are Racing to Make Weed as Easy to Drink as Beer." *Bloomberg*. February 6, 2019.

Powers, Deb. "How to Make CBD Cocktails at Home." *Civilized*. September 4, 2018.

Perucca, E. "Cannabinoids in the Treatment of Epilepsy: Hard Evidence at Last?" *Journal of Epilepsy Research*. December 2017.

Ross, Michelle N. *Vitamin Weed: A 4-Step Plan to Prevent and Reverse Endocannabinoid Deficiency*. Green Stone Books. 2018.

Russo, Dr. Ethan. "CBD, the Entourage Effect and the Microbiome." *Project CBD*. January 7, 2019.

Russo, Ethan. "Taming THC: Potential Cannabis Synergy and Phytocannabinoid-Terpenoid Entourage Effects." *British Journal of Pharmacology*. August 2011.

Salarizadeh, C. "Cannabis Consumer Behavior Alters with Covid-19 Quarantine: Edibles & Drinks Surge." *Green Market Report*. April 3, 2020.

Silvestro, S. et al. "Use of Cannabidiol in the Treatment of Epilepsy: Efficacy and Security in Clinical Trials." *Molecules*. April 24, 2019.

Staff Writer. "11-Hydroxy-THC—Increased Potency that Explains the Effect of Edibles?" *Prof of Pot*. July 2, 2019.

Weber. B., et al. *Cocktails Made Simple*. Emeryville, CA: Rockridge Press. 2019.

Welty, Timothy E., et al. "Cannabidiol: Promise and Pitfalls." American Epilepsy Society. September 2014–2015.

White, C. M. "A Review of Human Studies Assessing Cannabidiol's (CBD) Therapeutic Actions and Potential." *Journal of Clinical Pharmacology*. July 2019.

RESOURCES

CBD Isolates

CBDistillery 99%+ Pure CBDelicious
  Formulation Powder

CBDistillery 99+% Pure CBD Isolate
  Powder (Crystalline)

Sun-Grown Flower

Flower Co.

Flow Kana

Aloha Humboldt

Alpenglow Farms

Tinctures

Care By Design Sublingual Drops

Care By Design Hemp CBD Drops

Juna

Om Edibles

Humboldt Apothecary

Infused Drinks

Artet cannabis aperitif

D'Fleur infused beverages

House of Saka infused beverages

Hi-Fi Hops

Kikoko

Proposition Cocktail Co.

Sōmatik

Wünder

Infusion/Decarboxylation Devices

Ardent Nova

Ardent FX

LEVO II oil infusion device

**Ready-to-Use Gourmet Cannabis
Products**

Potli infused honey and apple cider
  vinegar

Pot d'Huile

Mondo Powder

Spirits & Liqueurs

Aperol

Hendrick's Gin

Bullet Rye Whiskey

Dolin Vermouth

Tres Agaves Tequila Blanco

Fidencio Mezcal Artesanal

Batiste Silver Rum

Timeless Vodka

Gifford Rhubarb Liqueur

St. George Dry Gin

St. Germain Elderflower Liqueur

Barsol Pisco

Three Sheets Spiced Rum

CANNABIS DRINKS

ACKNOWLEDGMENTS

First and foremost, I'd like to thank my mother, Nancy Evans, for helping me think of the concept before her passing in October 2019. She was so fascinated to learn more about cannabis-infused drinks and encouraged me to write this book covering these exotic elixirs. I'd also like to thank my father, Jim Evans, for his endless support and encouragement. I love you, Dad.

I want to thank my wonderful husband, Stratos Christianakis, for being my biggest cheerleader. Your love continues to inspire me. Thank you so much for all that you do, and thank you for sampling all of my recipes! I love you.

I'd like to thank my sister, Kayla, and brother-in-law, Mishka, for always believing in me. When times were really tough at the end of 2019, you were always there and encouraged me to write this book.

Thank you to my extended families, The Barbers, The Evanses, The Christianakises, and The vom Dorps, for your support and believing in my vision to write two cannabis books. I love you.

A heartfelt thank you to Quarto Publishing Group and Fair Winds Press for being the best publishing house to work with.

I want to thank my wonderful editor, Thom O'Hearn! I also want to thank my project manager, Meredith Quinn; art director, David Martinell; and Quarto's brilliant design team. This book is so beautiful. Also, a big shout out to my fantastic copyeditor, Jenna Patton. You rock!

A big thank you to my fabulous photographer and friend, Colleen Eversman of 2nd Truth Photography, who shot the incredible photos for this book. We did it!! Cheers to book #2!!

A heartfelt thank you to my wonderful cannabis and drink expert contributors including Cynthia Salarizadeh, Tracey Mason, Max Montrose, Maya Elisabeth, Jeremy Marshall, Felicity Chen, Christine Yi, Ben Larson, Dr. Harold Han, Christopher Schroeder, Clayton Coker, Erin Willis, Jewel Zimmer, Rachel Burkons, Warren Bobrow, and Tarita Noronha. You are all pioneers in this industry and I am beyond grateful for the information that you were willing to share. Cheers to the future of cannabis drinks!

Last but not least, I want to thank my wonderful fans and readers who've supported my work from the very beginning. I love you all and I am so grateful for this community.

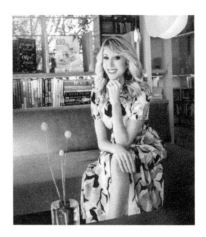

ABOUT THE AUTHOR

Jamie Evans is the founder of The Herb Somm, a culinary-meets-cannabis blog and lifestyle brand that is focused on the gourmet side of the industry. She is an author and entrepreneur specializing in cannabis, CBD, food, wine, and the canna-culinary world.

As a well-known CBD and cannabis personality, Jamie has contributed to *POPSUGAR, MARY Magazine*, and *The Clever Root* magazine specializing in cannabis and CBD lifestyle features for the modern consumer. She's also the co-editor of GoldLeaf's acclaimed cannabis *Cooking Journal* and author of *The Ultimate Guide to CBD: Explore the World of Cannabidiol* (Fair Winds Press).

As an industry leader, Jamie was named one of *Wine Enthusiast* magazine's Top 40 Under 40 Tastemakers in 2018 and as a 2018 Innovator by *SevenFifty Daily*, both recognizing her efforts in the cannabis industry. She was also recognized as one of *Green Market Report's* "Most Important Women in Weed" in 2020.

Alongside her work in the cannabis space, Jamie has over a decade of wine industry experience. As a Certified Specialist of Wine, she continues her wine education at the San Francisco Wine School.

The Herb Somm was created in March 2017 with the goal of educating consumers about healthy ways to incorporate herbal products into everyday life focusing on cannabis pairings, recipes, wellness, and CBD/cannabis education. Follow Jamie's canna-culinary adventures on Instagram and Twitter @theherbsomm.

INDEX

ALSO BY JAMIE EVANS

The Ultimate Guide to CBD

ISBN: 978-1-59233-926-6

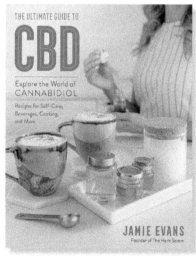

THE ULTIMATE GUIDE TO
CBD
Explore the World of CANNABIDIOL
Recipes for Self-Care, Beverages, Cooking, and More

JAMIE EVANS
Founder of The Herb Somm

Milton Keynes UK
Ingram Content Group UK Ltd.
UKHW051111150224
437754UK00010B/154